Intensive Care for Nurses

EDITED BY

D. B. CLARKE
MB FRCS

Consultant Cardiothoracic Surgeon
United Birmingham Hospitals

AND

A. D. BARNES
ChM FRCS

Consultant General and
Transplant Surgeon
United Birmingham Hospitals
Honorary Senior Lecturer in Surgery
University of Birmingham

THIRD EDITION

Blackwell Scientific Publications

OXFORD LONDON EDINBURGH
BOSTON MELBOURNE

© 1971, 1975, 1980
Blackwell Scientific Publications
Editorial offices:
Osney Mead, Oxford OX2 0EL
8 John Street, London WC1N 2ES
9 Forrest Road, Edinburgh EH1 2QH
52 Beacon Street, Boston,
　　Massachusetts 02108, USA
214 Berkeley Street, Carlton
　　Victoria 3053, Australia

First published 1971
Second edition 1975
Third edition 1980

Set in VIP Century Schoolbook
By Western Printing Services Ltd,
Bristol
Printed and bound in Great Britain by
Billing and Sons Ltd., Guildford,
London and Worcester.

Distributors

USA
　Blackwell Mosby Book
　Distributors
　11830 Westline Industrial Drive
　St. Louis, Missouri 63141

Canada
　Blackwell Mosby Book
　Distributors
　120 Melford Drive,
　Scarborough,
　Ontario M1B 2X4

Australia
　Blackwell Scientific Book
　Distributors
　214 Berkeley Street, Carlton
　Victoria 3053

British Library
Cataloguing in Publication Data

Intensive care for nurses. – 3rd ed.
　1. Intensive care nursing
　I. Clarke, David Barry
　II. Barnes, Anthony David
　616　　RT120.I5　　80–41315

　ISBN 0–632–00696–X

Contents

List of Contributors

D. B. Clarke, MB, FRCS
Consultant Cardiothoracic Surgeon, United Birmingham Hospitals.

A. D. Barnes, ChM., FRCS
Consultant General and Transplant Surgeon, United Birmingham Hospitals.
Honorary Senior Lecturer in Surgery, University of Birmingham.

B. L. Pentecost, MD, FRCP
Consultant Cardiologist, United Birmingham Hospitals.
Consultant-in-Charge, Coronary Care Unit, General Hospital, Birmingham.

J. McN. Inglis, MB, FFARCS
Consultant Anaesthetist, United Birmingham Hospitals.
Consultant-in-Charge, Intensive Care Unit, General Hospital, Birmingham.

Keith D. Roberts, ChM., FRCS
Consultant Cardiothoracic Surgeon, Birmingham Children's Hospital.
Clinical Director, Intensive Care Unit, Birmingham Children's Hospital.

Preface to the Third Edition

Advances in the treatment of very sick patients during the past decade have necessitated major alterations to the text of this edition. The general format remains the same. Biochemical and other values are now expressed in SI units with an introductory table of normal laboratory values. Basic nursing techniques are described adequately elsewhere. In this text we aim to supplement the knowledge of nurses employed in intensive care units of all types.

Preface to the First Edition

Stimulated by the development of open heart surgery, intensive care in Birmingham began in a converted examination room containing two standard hospital beds. Monitoring equipment was improvised in the research laboratories or adapted from standard apparatus. From these small beginnings has evolved the chain of intensive care units now functioning in the hospitals of the Birmingham teaching group; each caters for different aspects of the care of the seriously ill patient, but all have a superb standard of nursing care in common.

If credit for this development is to be given to any one person, it must surely be to the late Sister Marion Simpson through whose energy and devotion intensive care nursing here was nurtured in those early days, to become respected specialty of nursing which it is today. She compiled a loose-leaf folder describing standard procedures which has been distributed to many centres in this country; this still forms the basic text used in our training course.

This book is dedicated to Sister Simpson.

The editors are conscious that criticism may be justly levelled at a multiple-author book for nurses written entirely by doctors. The omission of a nursing contributor is no slight to that profession; it is indeed a tribute to the unique status of the intensive care nurse. It is assumed that the reader is well grounded in standard nursing techniques. She now moves into the hinterland between the medical and nursing professions where she will be required to exercise a degree of initiative and accept a measure of responsibility which is often greater than that expected of a newly qualified doctor. This must be rooted in an understanding of medicine, surgery and physiology which can best be explained by a specialist in those fields. No single contributor could have written the whole of this book; it is our hope that, together, we will provide not only a guide to the advanced care of the seriously ill, but also indicate some of the fundamental reasons underlying the various procedures.

At every step, the typescript has been subjected to the searching, but always friendly, criticism of our colleagues, the sisters in charge of the intensive care units of the United Birmingham Hospitals.*

We are grateful to them for their invaluable assistance in this, and also for their cheerful camaraderie and untiring support. Intensive care is worrying, tiring, often disheartening but always challenging and fascinating. Without our nursing colleagues, neither intensive care would have developed nor this book have been written.

---

* The authors are indebted to Miss Pauline Jones for her invaluable help in the typing of this manuscript.

Normal Laboratory Values (SI units)

Blood

Alkaline phosphatase	3–14 KA units
Ammonia	0.5–1.7 μgNH$_3$/ml
Amylase	<160 u/dl
B$_{12}$	140–900 pg/ml
Base excess	± 2.3 mmol/l
Bicarbonate (standard)	22–26 mmol/l
Bilirubin	3–21 μmol/l
Calcium	2.20–2.64 mmol/l
Chloride	95–105 mmol/l
Cholesterol	3.1–8.5 mmol/l
Cholinesterase (pseudo)	9–25 mol/ml/min
CPK	<130 iu/l
Creatinine—males	60–125 μmol/l
—females	45–110 μmol/l
Creatinine clearance	76–160 ml/min
Glucose	3.0–7.0 mmol/l
Haemoglobin—males	13.5–18.0 g/dl
—females	11.5–16.5 g/dl
PCV—males	40–54%
—females	35–47%
Lactic acid	0.5–2.0 mmol/l
LDH	120–365 iu/l
Magnesium	0.70–0.95 mmol/l
5 Nucleotidase	4–14 iu/l
Osmolarity	278–294 mmol/kg
PCO$_2$	4.7–6.0 kPa
H$^+$ (pH)	36–43 nmol/l
Phosphate	0.7–1.4 mmol/l
Platelets	150–400
PO$_2$	11.3–14.0 kPa
Potassium	3.4–5.1 mmol/l
Protein—total	63–79 g/l
—albumin	25–50 g/l
—globulin	18–30 g/l
Prothrombin time	10–14 seconds
Sodium	134–146 mmol/l

Thyroxine T_4	60–135 nmol/l
Transaminase SGOT	5–30 iu, μmol/l/min
SGPT	5–30 iu
Urea—males	2.7–12.3 mmol/l
—females	2.2–10.7 mmol/l
Volume (blood)	4–8l; 85 ml/kg body weight
White blood cells	4000–11 000

Values at individual hospitals may vary due to slight differences in technique. Staff should be aware of the normal range of their own laboratories.

Chapter 1
The Concept of Intensive Care

It is difficult to define an intensive care unit (ICU) but it is important to do so before entering the complexities of the subject.

The shortest definition as 'The place where the sickest patients are nursed' is pithy, but somewhat uninformative. More accurately, the intensive care unit could be defined as an area where seriously ill patients can be treated by the most highly qualified staff, under the best possible conditions with the most modern equipment within easy reach. A longer definition but more explicit.

Immediately, certain difficulties will become apparent. How is a patient to be classified as 'seriously ill'? Are all patients in danger of dying to be admitted to the unit? Obviously not. The compromise between the ideal and the often limited facilities available haunts hospital planners. Even the need for the most highly qualified nursing staff implies certain difficulties. How is such staff to be trained? Will the creation of a nursing élite to run the ICU be a disrupting influence to the running of the general wards? These problems must be recognized, and intensive care nursing is here to stay. Its worth to the patient has been demonstrated again and again. The management of the patient with coronary artery disease, the success of complicated surgery, indeed the practice of modern medicine would be sorely handicapped without intensive care units.

Design of the intensive care unit

While it may be possible to design a unit as an integral part of a new hospital, it is sometimes necessary to adapt some parts of an existing, often old-fashioned, hospital.

Siting is important, and must to some extent be dictated by the type of patient to be treated. If the unit will be mainly used for the care of the surgical patient, it is best sited near the operating theatre. If a more general range of disease is to be treated a central position may be more suitable. It is now accepted that a general hospital should have one intensive care bed for every hundred beds in the wards. If it also has units undertaking such demanding work as cardiac or transplantation surgery the provision of intensive care beds should be more generous.

The relationship between the size of the unit and the number of beds it contains requires careful consideration. Ample space between the beds is essential not only to accommodate bulky equipment, but also to allow easy access to the patient. Further, it is essential to have room between the head of the bed and the wall so that endotracheal intubation or bronchoscopy can be performed easily.

In units primarily concerned with respiratory problems it may be found that the practice of having the patient's head lying towards the centre of the ward will confer many advantages. Mechanical ventilators are certainly more easily accessible and tracheostomy care is facilitated.

Cross infection between patients in the unit is a problem. Its prevention should be considered in planning bed-spacing. There is much to be said for having two separate units—clean and dirty, so that patients known to have a potential source of infection such as a discharging wound sinus or pneumonia, can be segregated. It has been our custom to transfer patients from the clean to the dirty unit if they develop an infection. While this protects the other patients in the clean area, it certainly is not in the best interests of the patient so transferred to be exposed to infection from other patients. The provision of single rooms and barrier nursing facilities should be considered for the units dealing with infective or immunosuppressed patients.

This problem could be overcome by nursing each patient in the unit in isolation. This suffers from the defects so well known in any ward composed of many single or double rooms. Adequate supervision is not possible without a large increase in nursing staff, and expensive equipment may need to be duplicated. A compromise, which is, however, not without some disadvantages, is the use of partial cubicles. Beds are separated by glass partitions which serve to contain infection while allowing the patient to be observed from a central nursing station (Fig. 1).

Intensive care implies continuous observation; so the unit must be lighted constantly. Background illumination from ceiling fittings should be colour corrected so that minor degrees of cyanosis or jaundice can be seen at all times. In addition, small portable spotlights must be available to allow minor surgical procedures to be carried out.

Each bed space must have piped oxygen, nitrous oxide, a vacuum line, and an air line. Multiple power points of standard size are

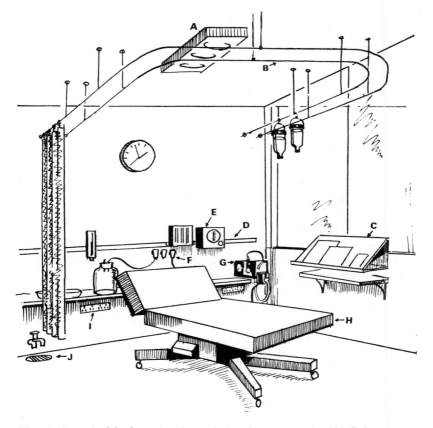

Fig. 1. A typical bed station in an intensive care unit. (A) Colour-corrected lighting; (B) overhead rail for suspending intravenous bottles; (C) desk for keeping records; (D) wall-mounted rail used to support equipment; (E) oscilloscope; (F) piped oxygen, air, suction and nitrous oxide; (G) mechanical ventilator; (H) intensive care unit bed; (I) multiple power points; (J) water supply and drain for use in renal dialysis.

essential. (13-amp ring main is the most satisfactory for general purposes but some modern dialysis machines require a 30 amp outlet.) Shelf space and a desk or work surface to support records and charts must be provided, adjacent to the bed. All surfaces must be able to withstand liquid germicides.

Much care and thought have gone into the design of the modern intensive care bed. The rails at head and foot have disappeared so that access to the patient from any quarter is unimpeded. The bed can be raised, lowered, or tilted, and its head can be raised so that the patient is propped in the sitting position. The base of the bed should be firm and translucent to X-rays. The mattress should be sufficiently firm to enable effective external cardiac compression to be performed; the spring mattress of a standard hospital bed is too soft for this purpose. Intravenous drip stands and oxygen cylinders should fix to the bed so that it is possible to wheel the patient about without a trailing procession of equipment. Latterly, rails mounted on the wall behind the bed have been introduced. Most equipment used in intensive care—such as suction reservoirs, trays and monitoring devices—may be supplied with special brackets which clamp onto the rail. Although the system is neat and flexible, a shelf is just as serviceable.

Cupboards and shelves for the many drugs and intravenous solutions needed must be conveniently sited within the unit. These substances and the equipment must be clearly labelled and stored in a logical position so that they are to hand in an emergency and their absence is obvious during stock taking.

The types of electronic and monitoring equipment needed will be dictated by the particular bias of the unit, but a defibrillator and some method of displaying the electrocardiogram and arterial blood pressure are essential. The complex field of mechanical support is considered fully in Chapter 5. It would be reasonable to provide one ventilator for each bed with an additional machine held in reserve for mechanical failure.

Minor procedures such as the insertion of an intravenous cannula or an intercostal tube will be carried out more speedily and efficiently if disposable sterile equipment and prepacked instruments are available. Equally important is a supply of sterile airways, endotracheal tubes, laryngoscopes and bronchoscopes so that respiratory obstruction can be relieved without delay. Ample space must be provided for the storage of this equipment.

Control of infection

Simple measures such as adequate space between beds and the segregation of infected patients provide the mainstay of infection control in most units. It is wise to regard the unit as an extension of the operating theatre; casual visiting should be discouraged and a high standard of cleanliness maintained. Regular checks by the bacteriology department will ensure that important foci of infection are not overlooked. The staff caring for patients in the 'dirty' unit should be rigidly excluded from the clean area, and should wear gowns, caps, masks and overshoes. This may have little practical effect in limiting infection, but the ritual of gowning certainly discourages casual visiting.

The rigid standards of asepsis so essential to the safe management of tracheotomies is described fully in Chapter 4.

While these elementary precautions are sufficient for units dealing with the usual variety of acute illness, they are certainly not enough for such specialized fields as the care of burns, or transplantation surgery. The practice of the reversed barrier nursing unit of the Royal Marsden Hospital at Sutton is an example of the superb standard of asepsis which can be achieved by obsessive attention to detail. This unit cares for patients with leukaemia who are being treated with cytotoxic drugs. As the ability of the body to resist infection is seriously impaired, every effort is made to exclude bacteria from the patients' environment.

The air to the individual cubicles is passed through fine filters which trap any particle greater than 0.5 μm. As it is blown into the room under positive pressure, it escapes under doors and through vents. The air is changed twenty times per hour. The use of extraction fans for ventilation has the opposite effect—air is sucked into the unit from outside corridors, bringing dirt and bacteria with it.

Bacteriostatic paint is used on walls, and the floors are coated with a sealing compound. Bedclothes are changed daily and not only laundered, but autoclaved.

Before nursing staff enter the unit they strip completely, wash with antiseptic soap and don sterile underwear and an Egyptian cotton blouse, trousers, gown, cap and mask. It was shown some years ago that showering promotes sweating which in turn increases bacterial contamination of the nurses' skin; showers are no longer part of the ritual.

No contaminated article is allowed to come into contact with the patient. Newspapers and books are baked and are passed into the unit through double-doored hatches. While in the hatch the articles are exposed to ultraviolet light which destroys most pathogens within 30 seconds. Even food is sterilized; considerable ingenuity is needed to ensure that food is palatable as well as germ-free. Salt and sugar are ̄gamma-ray sterilized, bread is rebaked, eggs are washed in hypochlorite solution, butter is autoclaved. Most tinned food is sterile, but precautions are taken to retain this sterility during serving. Crockery and utensils are autoclaved. Simple boiling eliminates most pathogens and this technique is used in the preparation of milk drinks, jellies and other foods. The ultimate culinary triumph is the preparation of a sterile birthday cake.

A second lock system is used to pass used crocks, bedpans and linen from the sterile to the service areas.

The efficiency of these precautions is regularly monitored by the bacteriology department; swabs are taken from the staff and culture plates are exposed in various parts of the unit at weekly intervals.

The isolation of the patient is made easier to bear by an intercom system—and, of course, by devoted nursing. The cubicles are cleaned between admissions with a synthetic phenol solution (Hycolin); all surfaces are saturated with a nebulizer.

This type of unit is very expensive to build and operate and at present has only a limited use. More recently plastic units have been designed so that single patients can be nursed in isolation. They can be installed relatively cheaply in an intensive care ward. They have the advantage that the staff can remain outside the isolator and perform most of the nursing procedures using gloves welded on to the sides of the unit. These units are likely to find application in the fields of burns, cytotoxic therapy and transplantation surgery.

Many of the lessons being learned in these most interesting projects may eventually be applied to the design and management of all intensive care units.

Qualifications for admission to the unit

It is much simpler to list those patients who are not suitable for intensive care than to define the requirements for admission.

The unit should not be used as a repository for the dying, even though terminal patient care may be demanding of both nursing and medical skill and time. This ruling may seem to be heartless, but must be followed if the morale of the unit is to be maintained. Nevertheless intensive care is such that mortality must inevitably be high. Nursing staff learn to accept this if the approach to patient care is one of positive optimism. The objective of restoring the patient, however ill, to health is a necessary spur. Success enables defeat to be more easily borne. If the resources of the unit are devoted to the care of the dying, morale suffers, recruitment of new staff will be impossible and the reputation of the unit as an ante-room to the mortuary will percolate through to patients in the ward awaiting surgery. Some units have failed to work satisfactorily because of this sort of abuse.

Equally important is the refusal to admit patients who require no more than standard nursing care. Pressure may be brought to secure the admission of patients solely for administrative convenience. A ward may be short-staffed or crowded, but the solution is not to be found in off-loading the additional work burden onto the unit. Neither must the unit staff be regarded as a nursing pool which can be tapped to supply deficiencies in the general hospital wards. The misuse of such specialized facilities is rather like using a chisel as a screwdriver. Inevitably, a line must be drawn between standard nursing care and intensive care. Such a division is bound to be arbitrary, but as a rough guide, the need for the attention of a nurse more often than once every half-hour will suffice.

A distinction must be made between treatment and observation. The care of a tracheostomy, the management of multiple injuries and burns are self-evident indications for intensive care. Equally valid is the need for frequent observation and recording in a patient who is not in extremis, but in whom there is a good chance of deterioration if changing signs are not noted and acted upon quickly. Proper observation is difficult in a main ward. The dim light, cramped conditions and fear of disturbing the other patients all hamper the nurse. Patients recovering from major thoracic and cardiac operations and those who have recently sustained head injuries certainly need such careful observation.

Frequent recordings of blood pressure are necessary after open heart surgery, trauma, and other major operations as more than fifteen minutes of hypotension can have far-reaching and often catastrophic side effects. The nurse in the ICU may be required to perform tasks such as bag and suck, blood sampling, intravenous injection and defibrillation not usually performed by nurses in the ordinary ward.

Finally, there is the role of the unit as a focus of special skills and experience in the management of certain specific diseases. The coronary care unit, the respiratory, burns and neurosurgical units, the sterile areas needed in some forms of transplantation surgery and cytotoxic therapy are representative of such special interests.

Staffing and responsibility

Paradoxically, so many doctors may have an interest in some aspect of the treatment that it is difficult to decide who is in overall charge of the patient. Some diplomacy may be necessary in order to avoid bruising sensibilities, and there are often occasions where tact and firmness must be combined.

The consultant under whom the patient was first admitted to the hospital is in a difficult position. He may have little to do with the routine running of the unit and he may feel that he has lost his special relationship with the patient by handing the responsibility to the unit personnel. Simple courtesy dictates that he should not be made to feel unwelcome. His suggestions and wishes should be noted, and the nurses can do much to ensure a friendly liaison between him and those managing the unit. At the same time, overall control must rest in one pair of hands. Contradictory instructions do little to help the patient. Some units prefer the referring consultant to order every stage of the treatment, others have a team working together, controlling every aspect of the running of the unit with a pool of experts in such fields as renal disease, psychiatry or neurology who can be consulted if necessary. The nurse must be in no doubt where to turn for help.

The acceptance of patients must be the responsibility of a doctor sufficiently senior to shoulder the sometimes difficult task of refusing the request of a consultant to admit his patient. He will be guided in making this decision by the criteria outlined above, by the number of vacant beds and availability of nursing staff. He has the further tasks of supervising the ordering of special equipment and controlling infection.

Intensive care cannot be effective if staffing falls lower than a ratio of one nurse to each patient throughout the 24 hours. Rather than compromise this principle it is better to restrict admissions during periods of nursing shortage. A high proportion of the staff should be staff nurses or sisters. If intensive care is entrusted to inexperienced, unsupervised nurses the standards of the unit will decline and the morale will fall. No nurse will want to continue to work in the unit and the constant turnover of staff will in turn affect recruitment. At a time when we are faced with a national shortage of nurses, this aspect presents the greatest threat to the furtherance of advanced medicine and surgery in this country. No easy solution exists, but surely an attempt to attract experienced part-time staff will help to ease the burden on the whole-time career nurses.

Fundamental observations in the very ill

The old tag 'Science is measurement' finds a new application in intensive care. In order to put the management of the seriously ill on a scientific footing, many variables are measured and recorded. Pulse, blood pressure and urine output, losses of blood, fluids and electrolytes, intravenous and oral fluid recordings, the electrocardiograph and a battery of biochemical investigations supplemented by X-rays, blood volume and sophisticated haemodynamic measurements ensure that every aspect of the patient's physical state is known. It is usual to take a radiograph of the chest each day. The ultimate in measurement is achieved in certain American centres where the computer has been harnessed to the patient. Variations in the recordings trigger off the appropriate blood replacement, administration of cardiac stimulant drug or even electrical defibrillation of the heart. Impressive as these advances may be, they in no way replace the trained nurse.

No computer yet made can look at a patient and judge whether he looks well or ill. No measurement, however delicate, can substitute for the instinct that all is not well which comes only from experience and careful observation. The first duty of the nurse is to look. Scientific aids should supplement observations not supplant them. On innumerable occasions, a change in facial expression, the appearance of a few beads of sweat, the onset of restlessness have warned of impending trouble long before 'the recordings' have altered. A slavish reliance on the impressive columns of figures on a balance chart is dangerous. Even if the volume of blood escaping from the drainage tubes after open heart surgery is recorded and charted every fifteen minutes, an assumption is made that every drop of blood lost from the vascular system finds its way to the underwater seal bottles. This may not always be so—we have seen two litres of blood collect in the chest because the tube had become blocked with clot. The recordings were perfect—every cubic centimetre of blood drained had been replaced by transfusion. A glance at the pale face and cold skin of the patient should have indicated that he was desperately short of blood.

Much information may be gained from simple observation. Observe the patient's general demeanour. The restless patient may be in pain or having difficulty in breathing. If a mechanical ventilator is being used, the patient should breathe with it. If he struggles, or attempts to remove the endotracheal tube, urgent action is needed to relieve his distress. Note the patient's level of consciousness and the way in which he responds to any nursing procedure. Does he cough when a suction catheter is passed into the trachea? Does he move his limbs equally well, or is one side paralysed or spastic?

Colour-corrected lighting enables the nurse to detect changes in skin colour with great accuracy. Cyanosis is most easily detected in the finger and toenails, the lips and tongue. Cultivate the habit of comparing the colour of your own nailbeds with those of the patient. As many patients will have indwelling arterial lines, the PaO_2 and $PaCO_2$ can be readily checked if there is any doubt. Jaundice is not infrequent after major surgery or trauma, and is usually not dangerous, but it may indicate the onset of liver failure. The yellowish tinge is first seen in the conjunctivae. Changes in the colour of urine in the closed drainage system should not be ignored. A deep orange tint is found in jaundice; pink or port wine red urine suggest haematuria or haemoglobinuria. The latter suggest the possibility of haemolysis as a result of trauma to the red cells by the heart-lung machine or an artificial heart valve or a mismatched blood transfusion.

Much can be learned from the feel of the patient's skin. The cold clamminess of circulatory failure and the hot flush of carbon dioxide poisoning are typical examples. In contrast to veterinary practice, a cold nose is not an indication of health, but rather of a low circulating blood volume. Become familiar with the normal elasticity of skin. If the patient is dehydrated a fold of skin pinched between finger and thumb remains standing up instead of springing back. The tongue may look and feel dry, but this sign will also be found in patients who breathe through the mouth. Learn to detect such early signs of oedema as the impression of your fingerprint on the skin or persistent circular depressions where a stethoscope has been applied to the chest. To detail every abnormality which can be detected by the trained eye would fill a very large book; increasing experience will be the best teacher of this vital aspect of clinical medicine. Careful observation is a habit which the intensive care nurse must cultivate assiduously.

Electronic equipment

There are few aspects of circulatory, respiratory, gastrointestinal and renal physiology which cannot be measured and recorded. Some of these measurements are excessively complicated, and can only be applied to experimental animals in the laboratory, but developments are such that several are finding their way into the ward. Although the nurse cannot be expected to understand the mathematics and complex electronics involved, she may be concerned with the routine management of equipment and will need to know something of the normal and abnormal values recorded. The significance of these values will be discussed later. It will suffice here to indicate the sort of recordings which may be obtained and to outline some of the principles which are involved.

Instruments which record naturally produced electrical currents generated within the body are essentially amplifiers. They are able to detect minute electrical impulses, to magnify them and then display them, either as a moving spot on a fluorescent screen or by moving a pen on a roll of paper. The most familiar examples are the electrocardiograph and the electroencephalograph. The controls of the bedside oscilloscope are simple. The luminous spot of light may be focused and its brightness may be increased or diminished. The knob marked Y axis moves the light spot up or down, so the ECG trace may be maintained in the middle of the screen. The speed at which the light spot travels across the screen may also be chosen. The uses of knobs which select the various electrocardiographic leads will be described in Chapter 3. Many oscilloscopes have an audible signal which emits a note with each heartbeat. Some instruments are capable of storing information so that the recordings can be played back. Others display a compressed recording so that changes and trends occurring over the course of several hours are seen readily.

The electrical thermometer is equipped with a probe with a tip which converts temperature changes into electrical impulses.

These move a spot of light or pointer along a calibrated scale or display figures. A method of monitoring the temperature continuously is of great value in the care of head injuries and the management of elderly patients suffering from cold and exposure (hypothermia).

Another group of instruments use pressure changes to modify an electric current (transducers or strain gauges). A diaphragm is moved by changes in pressure. This movement affects the resistance to the flow of a current through the transducer. The change in resistance in turn can be displayed on an oscilloscope screen or by a pen writer. The most useful application of the pressure transducer is in the continuous monitoring of the arterial pressure; less commonly the pressure in the right or left atrium may be recorded. A fine plastic cannula is inserted into an artery or vein and connected to the recorder. Of course, the cannula will clot unless it is continuously flushed with heparin (500 units in 500 ml of N. saline). Care must be taken to ensure that no air is allowed into the system, as not only will the accuracy of the recording be impaired, but air bubbles entering the left atrium or the arteries may find their way to the brain. Electrolyte solution in a plastic bag may be surrounded by an inflatable cuff. This is connected to the flushing system and the required pressure is obtained by blowing up the cuff. A slow, controlled flow of the solution is maintained by a valve which is incorporated in the system. If blood appears in the lines, as for example after withdrawing blood samples, rapid flushing is achieved by tugging on a rubber tag connected to the valve unit.

By applying a known pressure to the transducer, two standard pressures are displayed—zero and 100 mmHg. The zero value is obtained by opening the transducer to atmospheric pressure, and then using the Y axis knob to move the trace until it corresponds with the zero value on the scale marked on the oscilloscope screen. A mercury column, such as is found in a sphygmomanometer, is now connected to the transducer, and pumped up until the mercury touches 100 mmHg. The position of the trace on the oscilloscope is now adjusted until it corresponds to the 100 mark on the scale or the equivalent of a 100 mmHg test load may be applied electronically. Pressures can now be read off with confidence, but this calibration must be repeated from time to time to compensate for variations which may occur in the electrical equipment. If the recordings appear to show a fall in the blood pressure, first check that the cannula in the vessel is patent by flushing some fluid through it, and then check the calibration. Then take the necessary steps to treat the hypotension. A flattened arterial pressure trace may be due to partial obstruction of the intra-arterial catheter or to air bubbles in the system.

The sophisticated and delicate instruments which measure the flow of blood or gases normally will not be a nurse's responsibility, and are not in general use. The sort of information which they provide can be of great value—the cardiac output, the work done by the heart, the force of contraction of the ventricles and the resistance to blood flow in the peripheral vessels can all be calculated from a knowledge of blood flow and blood pressure. Hopefully, the future nurse will see the widespread use of these instruments. The sensitive probe which detects blood flow works in one of three ways. It may detect the changes in a magnetic field applied across a blood vessel, or the rate at which heat is dissipated by the passage of blood, or it may utilize the Doppler effects. This is most familiar as the change in pitch of a train whistle as it first approaches and then recedes from you. The Doppler flow probe projects a beam of ultrasound across the vessel which is reflected by the solid elements in the bloodstream. A 'change in pitch' occurs and is varied by the speed with which these solid particles move. The thermal technique uses a catheter probe which is sensitive to temperature changes. Cold fluid is injected upstream from this probe and the changes in blood temperature so produced are measured. The degree to which the blood is cooled is proportional to the speed at which it is flowing.

The cardiac output may be estimated by injecting a known quantity of dye into a vein and then withdrawing blood from an artery at a constant rate. The blood is passed through an instrument which detects the dye as it appears in the arterial blood. It is possible to calculate the cardiac output from estimations of how rapidly the concentration of dye builds up in the sample withdrawn, but the mathematics are complicated, and a small computer is built into the machine to work out the answers.

The principle of measuring the dilution of a known volume of a substance injected into the bloodstream is used to calculate the volume of blood in the body—the substances used are either a dye or radioactive albumin. The value of such measurements in caring for a patient who is bleeding is obvious, but there are drawbacks which are discussed in Chapter 2. Much useful information can also be derived from simple observation and measurement of arterial and venous pressures.

This all sounds very technical and complicated, and of course blood volume and cardiac output measurements require specialized medical knowledge. However, the time may not be too far distant when methods will have been simplified to a point where the intensive care nurse will be able to handle them with confidence.

Electrical equipment, such as cardiac defibrillators and cardiac pacemakers will be described in Chapter 3.

A note of caution must be sounded. The electrolyte solutions and blood in intravenous and intra arterial cannulae conduct electricity—and the patient is often surrounded by and connected to electrical equipment. An electrical current too small to be felt by a hand on the patient's skin may be enough to provoke a fatal cardiac arrythmia. It is important that all electrical equipment is carefully maintained and safely earthed individually.

Biochemical and haematological measurement

Any one of the vast range of estimations which are performed in the biochemical and haematological laboratories may be needed, but a certain number of basic measurements should be performed every day to monitor the general progress of the patient's illness. These are the urine and serum electrolytes and urea, to confirm that the fluid and electrolyte needs of the patient are being supplied and that the kidneys are functioning properly, the haemoglobin and possibly the red and white cell counts, and the levels of carbon dioxide, the pH and sodium bicarbonate in the blood. The latter are essential information if the patient is being treated with a mechanical ventilator, and will often be supplemented by estimation of the oxygen content (PO_2) of a specimen of arterial blood.* The significance of these measurements is discussed in Chapters 4 and 6.

Effect of intensive care on the nurse

It is not my intention to compile a list of desirable characteristics for the ideal nurse, still less to offer advice as to conduct and

---

* The commonly used PO_2 is used throughout rather than the more correct PaO_2 of the physiologist.

bearing, but it must be said that intensive care nursing demands something special. The work is not to everyone's taste—the constant succession of emergencies, the frequent failures, the feeling that just as the patient is becoming sufficiently well to respond to his nurses and to appreciate all that is being done for him he is returned to the ward, all conspire to make the atmosphere a little impersonal. Not every nurse can shoulder the additional responsibility; some find the air of crisis, the complicated equipment and the rather high powered treatment frightening. Again, there is sometimes a feeling that nurses working in the general wards regard the unit nurses as 'different'. But for the woman or man who is able to overcome all these difficulties, there can be no more exciting or interesting work. The nurse is in the forefront of medical development and playing a vital part.

A cheerful, even informal atmosphere maintains morale and relieves the tension within the unit, provided it is always understood that the nurses' common sense and self-discipline will never allow this to degenerate into a slipshod or lackadaisical attitude. The nurse is part of a team, and should never feel shy about pointing out signs which she has observed or giving her opinion about the patient's progress and the effect of treatment. We are trying to treat patients efficiently, using every laboratory and scientific aid to define his illness precisely and scientifically. So there is no place for vague replies like 'He's as well as can be expected' when the nurse is asked how the patient is. I can best illustrate the sort of approach to be encouraged by recording the following. It was late at night, and I phoned the unit to enquire about a patient who had had a major cardiac operation earlier in the day. A staff nurse answered 'he's sleeping comfortably, tolerating his ventilator well with a minute volume of 10 litres. The blood pressure is steady at 110 systolic, the pulse rate is 90, with no pulse deficit. The total blood loss so far is 400 ml, but he is only draining about 10 cc every 15 minutes and the venous pressure is 10, so we've got the blood volume right.

'He's warm and pink, putting out about 30 ml of urine an hour. Oh, I've just noticed that the T waves on the electrocardiograph are getting a bit tall, so I've reduced the amount of potassium in the drip.'

Perfect!

Chapter 2
Maintaining an Adequate Circulation

A glance into any motoring magazine will reveal a bewildering number of different ways of describing the performance of a car. Such terms as capacity, brake horsepower and revolutions per minute confuse the uninitiated. However, any housewife can drive her car to the shops with the basic knowledge that there is petrol in the tank, that the battery is charged and how to start the engine. Looking after a patient's circulation is very similar to this.

The function of the heart may be described very precisely. It is possible to measure the volume of blood which it is pumping, the pressures in all its chambers, and the amount of work which it has to do if one has enough expertise and a lot of very expensive equipment, but all that is required of the nurse is that she should be able to answer two simple questions. Has the patient an adequate volume of blood in his circulatory system? Is the heart pumping that blood round efficiently? These questions are absolutely fundamental and it is possible to answer them by using observation aided by a few simple measurements. Of course, everyone is familiar with the picture of a patient who is bleeding to death, dead white, with a cold sweaty skin. The pulse is flickering and difficult to feel and the blood pressure may be unrecordable. If the patient is young and fit, he may even now be saved by prompt and rapid blood transfusion but the same order of blood loss in a patient, who for example, has just had a major heart operation would be very poorly tolerated, and would almost certainly lead to death. The point must again be made that the object of intensive care is as much to prevent troubles developing as to treat desperate emergencies. Early recognition of the failing heart, the reduced circulating blood volume, the inadequately oxygenated patient and the patient developing disturbances of his water and electrolyte balance is extremely important. Once matters have been allowed to advance to a state where the patient's plight can be recognized by anybody as they walk through the door of the unit, the point of no return has probably been passed. The patient accepted for intensive care is living on a knife-edge. If one of his physiological systems is allowed to go wrong the effect will reverberate around the other systems in the body. For example, if a patient is allowed to become hypoxic the heart will fail and as the circulation is impaired the kidneys will fail. It is rather like building a card house and then pulling the bottom card out. Let us now look a little more closely into the way that the two questions posed above can be answered.

Has the patient an adequate blood volume?

In a normal adult patient the circulatory system contains about 5 litres of blood, or 70–100 ml per kg of body weight. About a third of this is contained within the arteries and the other two-thirds is in the thinner walled and more distensible veins. A healthy person is able to lose one or two pints of blood without any serious effects. The body compensates for this loss of blood in several ways. Blood is diverted from less important areas such as the skin and the bowel to the vital centres such as the brain and the kidney. The blood vessels in these less important areas constrict and this is why the skin becomes pale and feels cold. The heart beats faster and the patient usually feels that he wants to lie down; this assists the circulation to the brain. The blood volume is restored to normal quite rapidly by fluid in the extracellular spaces passing into the vascular bed and in the course of the following days the lost red blood corpuscles and white blood corpuscles are replaced by the bone marrow. If the haemoglobin of a patient who has lost a pint of blood is estimated, the early readings will be normal, then a little later as the blood is diluted by fluid passing in from the extravascular spaces the haemoglobin level will fall. In the following days it will gradually return to normal again. It is therefore necessary to know first whether the patient is bleeding, secondly, how much blood he has lost and thirdly, if the amount of blood he is being given by transfusion is sufficient to bring the blood volume back to normal.

Clinical assessment of hypovolaemia

If blood loss is occurring into the bowel or a similar site where it cannot be detected easily, it is necessary to rely on physical signs to determine whether the blood volume is reduced. These signs are a rising pulse rate, pale cold skin and in the later stages, a falling blood pressure. It should be remembered that a young person can compensate for blood loss so efficiently that the blood pressure may sometimes rise. There are some situations where it is possible to make a more accurate assessment of the amount of blood lost. It has been calculated by measuring the girth of the thigh of patients with a fractured femur that such an injury results in the loss of about 1500 ml of blood into the spaces between the muscles and similar estimations have been made for most of the other common fracture sites (Fig. 2). Hence, if the patient has multiple injuries it is possible to count the number of fractures and calculate the amount of blood which has therefore been lost from the circulation.

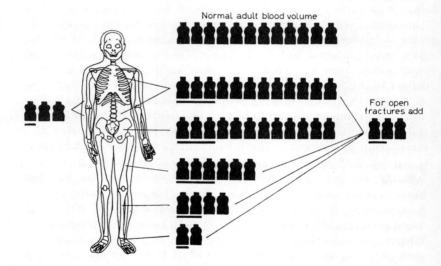

Fig. 2. The need for blood is indicated by the nature of the injury. The person illustrated is assumed to have a normal blood volume of about 5 litres, which is the amount of blood contained in 12 bottles of blood. The bottles underlined in each row indicate the usual order of loss; the entire row indicates the loss that may have to be made good in severe closed injuries. When there is an open fracture the need for blood is further increased.

From *Nursing Emergencies* (Blackwell 1967) with acknowledgements to Mr. P. S. London.

Probably quite a lot more is hidden away in body cavities as a result of internal injury. A further cause of a diminished blood volume is found after severe burns with extensive loss of skin. The raw areas weep copious amounts of protein-rich serum; and quite large volumes of blood may also be lost as a result of charring of muscle and other soft tissues. These losses must be made good by transfusion of either whole blood or plasma.

Direct measurement of blood losses

The patient who has undergone cardiac or pulmonary surgery is usually returned to the unit with drainage tubes in the pericardium or the pleural spaces which are connected to underwater seal bottles. We use large measuring cylinders for this purpose so that the volume of blood loss can be measured accurately. Every quarter of an hour the nurse records the volume of blood that has collected in the measuring cylinder and compares this with the volume of blood that has been given by transfusion. It would therefore seem that if every drop of blood which was drained was replaced by an equal volume of transfused blood, that the patient's blood volume could be kept to a steady normal level and post-operative care would then be simply a matter of tidy book-keeping. We certainly make a practice of measuring blood losses regularly and using this as a guide to replacement, but at the same time we recognize that the method has fallacies and that commonsense must be used. It is very easy to blind oneself into thinking that careful measurement and meticulous recordings are scientific and hence infallible but unfortunately such is not the case. Tubes may become blocked or the bleeding may be into undrained areas. It has been estimated that as much as a litre of blood can be infiltrated into the tissue planes of the mediastinum after heart surgery and this will certainly never find its way down a drainage tube. It is therefore necessary to take the patient's general condition into consideration when assessing blood loss.

Estimation of the circulating blood volume

Simple observation is valuable. If the patient is pale with blanching of the lips, lobes of the ears and nailbeds, suspect that he may be short of blood. A rising pulse rate and a falling systolic blood pressure also indicates hypovolaemia: the significance of these will be discussed more fully below. Direct estimations of the blood volume may be made by techniques involving the measurement of the degree of dilution of an injected sample of either dye or radioactive material. They are not commonly performed as they are not very accurate and in a changing clinical situation are of less clinical value than observations of fluid balance, blood pressure, pulse rate, central venous pressure recordings and the general clinical state of the patient.

Central venous pressure

If the blood pressure in an artery in the head and in the foot is measured, the results obtained will be quite similar. The veins, however, respond rather differently. In the standing position the pressure in the veins will be different when measured above and below the heart. At the level of the right atrium of the heart, the pressure is about 0–5 cm of water. The pressure in the feet would be much higher were it not for the venous valves. In fact it is the pressure which would be recorded at the bottom of a length of glass tubing as high as the distance between the heart and the ground if it was filled with water. The pressure in the veins on top of the head would have a negative value. If you sit on the edge of the bed with your feet dangling over the side, you will notice that the veins on the dorsum of the foot are distended and tense. If you lie down with your feet in the air the veins will rapidly empty. Therefore, the pressure in a vein is directly related to its position relative to the heart. The central venous pressure is an estimate of the pressure in the right atrium of the heart. It is possible to introduce a fine catheter into the right atrium by way of a peripheral vein and measure the pressure there directly with a simple water manometer. The same result may be obtained indirectly by recording the pressure in any peripheral vein with a water manometer and relating the height of the column of liquid in the manometer to the level of the heart. We usually take the manubriosternal junction as being approximately the level of the right atrium. Some people prefer to use a point in the patient's mid-axillary line. Various factors may influence the pressures recorded. As the patient breathes in and out the pressure level will be seen to rise and fall. If the lungs are being inflated by a mechanical ventilator, the pressure will rise; if the heart fails so that blood is dammed back in the venous system, the pressure will rise. If the blood volume is low, then the pressure will fall and it is its value in this regard that must now be considered.

How to measure the central venous pressure

A long intravenous catheter is inserted into a peripheral vein; the most convenient is the external jugular vein or, by using a cut down technique, the long saphenous vein may be used, but as stated above any cannula in a peripheral vein will do. In recent years doctors have become skilled at passing cannulae into the internal jugular or subclavian veins by direct puncture through the skin. This technique ensures reliable and long-term recording, and also provides a central line down which inotropic drugs can be given safely. The cannula is attached to an intravenous drip with a three-way tap in the line. A length of drip extension tubing is now inserted into the side arm of the three-way tap and filled with clear fluid from the drip bottle. The tap is now turned so that the tubing communicates with the cannula in the vein and the level of fluid will fall until it reaches a steady level. Hold the tubing so that a length of it is vertically over the manubriosternal junction and measure the height of the fluid column in centimetres with a ruler. Having taken the measurement, turn the three-way tap so that the drip runs slowly to prevent the cannula from clotting (Fig. 3).

More conveniently, the pressure may be measured with a transducer and displayed on an oscilloscope. The transducer must be kept level with the manubriosternal junction. We have found it convenient to stick it to the anterior chest wall with an adhesive pad. A system to flush the cannula continuously is essential.

Interpretation of the central venous pressure

It is wrong to consider the central venous pressure as being like the fuel gauge of a car. It does not record the number of pints of blood in circulation. It merely tells you whether the vascular compartment is full of blood, whether it is depleted or whether it is over-full. If the venous pressure is low, then the patient probably has a low blood volume. If it is high this usually indicates cardiac failure or cardiac tamponade. Some difficulty is encountered where the pressure is of the order of about 10–15 cm of water. It is then difficult to decide whether the patient is in cardiac failure or possibly has cardiac failure combined with hypovolaemia. A rapid infusion of about 100 ml of blood will usually provide the answer. If the patient has a low blood volume his circulatory state will improve and the blood pressure will rise, but the venous pressure will remain unchanged. If, however, he is in cardiac failure, the venous pressure will rise without any corresponding improvement in the circulation. Note that vasodilation also lowers the venous pressure because the blood volume no longer fills the expanded vascular bed. The effect is the same as a serious haemorrhage.

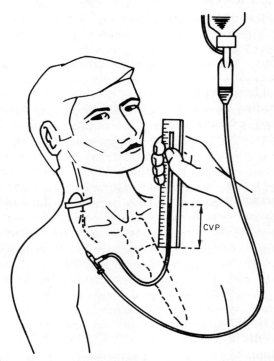

Fig. 3. Measuring central venous pressure. The central venous pressure is equivalent to the height of the column of liquid in the side arm above the manubriosternal junction.

Treatment of hypovolaemia

There is no doubt that the best replacement for lost blood is a blood transfusion. It is not my purpose to attempt to describe the complex field of cross-matching and blood grouping but there are certain practical features which will concern the nurse directly. First, how fast may blood be given? There is a popular misconception that giving blood rapidly may precipitate heart failure. It may certainly do so if the patient's blood volume is normal and if he is on the verge of heart failure, but the central venous pressure will provide an invaluable guide. If the patient has a low blood volume the heart cannot be expected to function efficiently. It may have difficulty in maintaining its own coronary circulation. No time should be lost in restoring the blood volume to normal but the nurse should be aware of the danger of giving a large volume of blood very rapidly. Stored blood is cold and rich in potassium. Effective devices for warming the blood are available, but a blood warmer may be improvised from a long coil of drip tubing immersed in a bucket of water at 37–40°C. The rate of the drip may be increased by elevating the drip stand or, if this is not sufficient, it may be pumped in under pressure with a compressible ball valve dripchamber, a Martin's pump attached to the drip tubing or, under medical supervision, air may be pumped into the bottle by a syringe attached to the air line. If this method is used, caution must be exercised as it is possible for the bottle to empty and for air to be pumped into the venous system under pressure. A very safe and satisfactory method is available when the blood is provided in polythene bags. These may be squeezed in an inflatable cuff which fits round the outside of the bag. Give the blood at a rate to replace the measured losses and to maintain the venous pressure at an acceptable level. It is useful to remember that a drip running at 30 drops a minute will deliver 500 ml of blood or clear fluid in 6 hours. If the drip fails to run there may be a number of manoeuvres that the nurse can try before calling for help. Of course, if a rapidly expanding swelling is seen at the site of the cannula, this means that the needle or cannula has come out of the vein and the drip must be stopped immediately. If no such swelling is seen, it is possible that the rapid infusion of cold blood has caused the vein to go into spasm. A warm pad on the arm may help. Sometimes the tip of a cannula jams against the side wall of the vein. All that is necessary is to withdraw it a few millimetres. A common cause of a drip stopping is that fluid has run into the air line and soaked the little plug of cotton wool, thereby effectively preventing any air from entering the bottle. When this happens the drip chamber will be seen to be collapsed. This is easily remedied by inserting a new air line. Nowadays most intravenous fluids are packed in plastic bags so that this problem does not occur.

Never forget that, no matter how desperate the emergency, blood must be carefully checked to make sure that the patient is not being given an incompatible transfusion. Discard any bag in which the supernatant plasma has a reddish tinge. This is found in old blood where there has been haemolysis of the red blood cells. Increasingly the blood transfusion service is producing blood component fractions for transfusion, so that the patient can get what he really needs—red cells, white cells, platelets and globulin, fresh frozen plasma, cyroprecipitated plasma, plasma protein fraction (PPF) etc. All blood donations are checked for the presence of hepatitis B antigen so post transfusion hepatitis is now extremely rare.

Clear fluids

Saline and dextrose solutions have little place in the management of a low circulating blood volume due to whole blood loss except under conditions of extreme urgency when no other fluid is available. Such fluids pass rapidly from the vascular bed into the extracellular compartment. Note that if dextrose is given into the same drip line as blood, clumps of red cells will be formed.

Plasma protein fraction (PPF)

Plasma is no longer available for infusion and has been replaced by PPF. This may be given for the same purpose as the previously available powdered plasma. PPF finds its greatest application in the treatment of burns. As much as half a litre may be lost in an hour in an extensively burnt adult. The amount to be infused is calculated from an estimate of the area of the burn expressed as a percentage of the total body surface and additional guidance is obtained by frequent measurements of the haematocrit. A rough guide to surface area divides the body into multiples of 9%. The head and arms each represent 9% of the total surface area. The front and back of the trunk account for 18% each and one leg represents 18%. The area of the palm of your hand is equivalent to 1%. As mentioned above, there may also be considerable red blood cell loss which will require blood for its replacement. Under emergency conditions it may be stated that a patient over 10 years of age will lose approximately 1–1½ litres of PPF for every 10% of the body surface which has been burned. Under 10 years of age an amount of plasma equal to the normal plasma volume for the patient is required for every 15% of the body surface burned. These amounts are the total plasma requirements, half of which should be given in the first 8 hours and the other half over the succeeding 16–24 hours. Another régime gives 110 ml of plasma and saline for every 1% of the body surface area burned in the first 48 hours. These are only rough guides and a far more accurate estimate can be made by the medical staff with the aid of nomograms.

Plasma substitutes

There are a variety of synthetic substitutes for plasma, with differing molecular weights. Dextran 40, 70, 90 and 120 are the most commonly encountered examples. They have the advantage that they are readily available and do not cause hepatitis but they make subsequent cross-matching of blood difficult and a specimen of blood must always be taken for this purpose before the infusion is commenced. They may also produce agglutination of the blood which on rare occasions may be fatal. Low-molecular-weight dextran is said to improve the circulation of blood in the capillaries; it appears to do this partly by attracting fluid into the vascular compartment and thereby reducing the viscosity of the blood.

Conditions predisposing to bleeding

Although full consideration of the diseases producing disorders of the clotting mechanism is beyond the scope of this book, there are certain conditions of which the nurse should be aware. It must first be appreciated that continued severe bleeding which requires massive blood replacement will eventually lead to a state where the blood no longer clots. This is partly because of the anticoagulant which is added to bank blood but also because stored blood is deficient in some of the vital clotting factors. There is a group of diseases, including haemophilia and Christmas disease, where bleeding is combated by fresh frozen plasma and infusions of anti-haemophilic globulin (AHG). Nowadays it is often possible to define the deficiency and give just that factor—platelets, AHG, etc. After open heart surgery the clotting mechanism may be disturbed in a variety of ways. Heparin is given during the operation to prevent coagulation of blood in the heart-lung machine. After the bypass is discontinued the heparin is neutralized by an appropriate amount of protamine, but sometimes the neutralization is not complete and further doses may be needed in the intensive care unit. Rarely, the patients may have enzymes in the blood which dissolve the fibrin in clots (fibrinolysins). This disorder is detected by incubating a specimen of clotted blood for a time and observing that the clot slowly dissolves. The syndrome of disseminated intravascular coagulation (DIC) is usually treated with several doses of heparin.

Is the heart functioning efficiently?—cardiac failure

Having discussed the role of a low circulating blood volume in circulatory failure, we must now consider failure of the pump itself. Cardiac failure may be due to hypoxia, in which the efficiency of the heart is impaired because it cannot work without oxygenated blood. Failure may also be due to disease and cardiac surgery, not only because the heart has been handled, but because patients who have needed valve replacement usually have a diseased and strained myocardium. Certain cardiac arrhythmias, in which the heart beats very quickly, will produce cardiac failure because there is not enough time between the rapid contractions of the ventricles to allow the heart to fill.

A normal person is able to increase the output of the heart in response to the demands of exercise without any rise in the pressures in the right and left atria. With mild degrees of heart failure an increased cardiac output may be achieved but only by an elevation of the pressure in these two atria. In severe heart failure a high atrial pressure is required to maintain an adequate cardiac output at rest. The elevation in pressure in these two atria is reflected back into the systemic and pulmonary veins. An elevated right atrial pressure produces a raised pressure in the great veins and this can be seen as distension of the jugular vein in the neck and by enlargement of the liver; these observations can be confirmed by measuring the central venous pressure (Fig. 4).

Oedema

Fluid is forced out of the vessels into the tissues, producing oedema of the legs and the back and collections of fluid in the peritoneal cavity (ascites). This is because the volume of fluid in the blood vessels is determined by a tug-of-war between two factors. On the one hand, forcing fluid out of the vessels, is the pressure in the capillaries and the veins. The osmotic pressure exerted by the proteins in the blood tends to hold the fluid in the blood vessels.

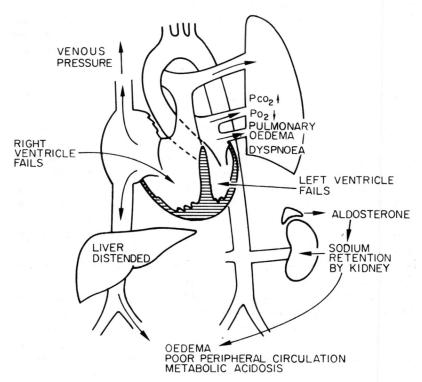

VENOUS
PRESSURE

P_{CO_2}
P_{O_2}
PULMONARY
OEDEMA
DYSPNOEA

RIGHT
VENTRICLE
FAILS

LEFT VENTRICLE
FAILS

ALDOSTERONE

LIVER
DISTENDED

SODIUM
RETENTION
BY KIDNEY

OEDEMA
POOR PERIPHERAL CIRCULATION
METABOLIC ACIDOSIS

Fig. 4. Diagram showing the effects of failure of the right and left ventricles.

Once the venous pressure rises the balance is upset and fluid is forced out into the tissues. The same mechanism operates on the left side of the heart where an elevation in the left atrial pressure also elevates the pressure in the pulmonary veins and this drives fluid out into the tissue spaces in the lungs, which become stiffer, and the patient complains of breathlessness. The aveoli may become filled with frothy fluid and the patient develops pulmonary oedema.

Failure of tissue perfusion

In addition to these back pressure effects from the failing heart, there are also serious consequences resulting from reduced blood flow to the body. Under-perfused tissues produce acid waste products. This metabolic acidosis in turn depresses the myocardium. Blood flow to the intestines falls to a third of normal levels and the kidney blood flow may be reduced by up to 75%. The reduced blood pressure in the kidney stimulates secretion of the hormone aldosterone by the adrenals, and this in turn forces the kidney to retain sodium.

Retention of sodium has two effects. The body counters the tendency for its fluids to become too salty (hypertonic) by retaining water and this retention of water will accentuate the production of oedema. The excess sodium will also tend to pass into the cells and as sodium passes in so potassium is forced out. Normally most of the body's potassium is found inside the cells and the sodium is found in the extracellular fluids. If the position of these two ions is reversed the function of the cell will be interfered with very profoundly and amongst the cells so affected are those comprising heart muscle, so that this in turn will tend to aggravate cardiac failure.

One of the body's natural responses to trauma and surgical operations is to produce aldosterone and also the antidiuretic hormone of the pituitary, again encouraging the retention of water and sodium. One disaster will rapidly compound another and heart failure with its far-reaching effects on all the body systems will rapidly enter a vicious spiral leading to the patient's deterioration and eventual death. Early recognition and prompt treatment is essential.

Recognition of heart failure

Ultimately, the most useful estimate of the function of the heart is measurement of cardiac output; that is, the volume of blood pumped by the heart in a minute. The output of the right ventricle must be the same as the output of the left ventricle otherwise all the blood would eventually collect in either the pulmonary or systemic circulations. The only exception to this rule is when there is some form of shunting between the right and left sides of the heart through a congenital defect in the interventricular or interatrial septum. The cardiac output at rest is of the order of 5 litres a minute and this may rise to 20 litres or more on exercise. You can imagine a tap filling an ordinary household bucket in a minute and you will have a conception of the volume of blood moved by the heart during light activities. Unfortunately, it is not easy to measure the cardiac output directly. The methods available are rather complicated and usually rely on injecting a sample of dye into the venous side of the circulation and then withdrawing a sample at a steady rate from the arterial side. The concentration of the dye is detected automatically by a photoelectric cell and then a small computer is used to calculate the cardiac output from the information thus obtained. Alternatively, the oxygen saturation in the right atrium and the arterial blood is determined while the patient breathes in and out of a spirometer. This instrument shows the amount of oxygen taken up by the lungs. From a knowledge of how much oxygen is picked up by the blood as it passes through the lungs, together with the volume of oxygen used in respiration in the course of a minute, the volume of blood passing through the lungs can be calculated (the Fick method). This represents the output of the right ventricle which, as we have said, is the same as the output of the left ventricle. It would be impracticable to make such complicated measurements very frequently and so we must rely on more indirect methods for assessing the performance of the heart.

Observation

If a patient's circulation is adequate, he will have a good colour, his fingers and toes will be warm and pink and the veins on the back of the hands and the dorsum of the foot will be full. If you milk such a vein empty with your finger it will be seen to fill again rapidly. The patient will breathe comfortably and the urine output will be at least of the order of 30 ml per hour. Contrast this with a patient in cardiac failure. The fingers and toes are blue and cold because blood has been diverted to more important centres. The neck veins may be distended and this is confirmed by estimating the central venous pressure, as described above. The skin is sometimes moist with sweat. Breathing is difficult because of pulmonary oedema and the patient may cough up frothy pink sputum or this may be aspirated from the endotracheal tube or tracheostomy. If a mechanical ventilator is being used, increasingly high pressures will be needed to maintain adequate respiratory volumes. This is because the machine is having to inflate lungs which are becoming progressively stiffer. A stethoscope will detect moist sounds over the bases of the lungs and the chest X-ray will reveal fluffy shadows over both lung fields.

It may be possible to recognize oedema, but if the patient is lying down it may not necessarily collect in the ankles. It may also be seen over the sacrum and behind the elbows. Oedema may be recognized by pressing the patient's skin firmly with the thumb and producing an impression or dent which slowly disappears. If the cardiac output continues to fall the legs will assume a blotchy blue and white mottled appearance and the patient will become increasingly drowsy and eventually unconscious.

The blood pressure

The pressure in the arteries depends upon two factors, the cardiac output and the peripheral resistance. The peripheral resistance is the resistance against which the heart has to pump and it depends upon the degree of constriction or dilation of the small arteries and capillaries. With every heartbeat the pressure rises to a high point (the systolic pressure) and between beats it falls to a low point (the diastolic pressure). The diastolic pressure too, is influenced by several factors, notably aortic incompetence, and changes in the peripheral resistance. A healthy heart in a young adult produces a blood pressure of about 120/80 and this pressure tends to rise with increasing age. The difference between the systolic and diastolic pressures is referred to as the pulse pressure. If the heart fails this difference will narrow so that recordings of the order of 110/90 will be obtained and it will become difficult to feel the pulse at the wrist. Whether the circulation is deteriorating because of cardiac failure or a low circulating blood volume, blood pressure will tend to fall. If it is allowed to reach levels of the order of 60 mmHg and to remain there, severe damage may be done to the kidneys (acute tubular necrosis) and as the circulation to the coronary arteries will be inadequate at these pressures heart failure will be further aggravated. Very ill patients, and patients who are the subject of particular concern after major surgery should have their blood pressures recorded every 15 minutes so that hypotension will be quickly recognized and corrected before irreversible damage has been done.

Measurement of the blood pressure (Fig. 5)

One of the most important skills which the intensive care nurse has to acquire is the ability to record the blood pressure accurately and to know when to call for help because it is abnormally low. A few practical points are worthy of note. If the patient is returned to the unit with an indwelling cannula in an artery and this is used to display the blood pressure on an oscilloscope screen, the matter is made simple and the nurse's sole responsibility is to ensure that the apparatus for flushing out the cannula to prevent clotting is kept in working order. However, most patients will have their blood pressures recorded with a sphygmomanometer. A cuff is placed firmly round the upper arm and inflated to a point at which the flow of blood down the brachial artery is obstructed. The pressure in the cuff, which is registered on a mercury manometer, must then be the same as the pressure in the artery. The point as which the flow of blood is just obstructed may be recognized by palpating the pulse at the wrist or the elbow and noting the point at which it just disappears, or more accurately, with the aid of a stethoscope. Mark the position of the brachial pulse, which is best felt just medial to the tendon of the biceps muscle, and place the stethoscope over this point. Inflate the cuff, and as it is allowed to deflate slowly, notice the pressure at which you first hear the sounds of the beating pulse. This is the systolic pressure. As the cuff is allowed to deflate further, these sounds will either disappear or suddenly become softer or muffled. The point at which they do this is the diastolic pressure. While this is an easy estimation to make in a healthy person, it can sometimes be difficult in patients with a low blood pressure, especially if they have had a previous cardiac catheterization or arteriogram which may have produced narrowing of the brachial artery. Under these circumstances, it is sometimes easier to record the blood pressure by palpating the pulse than with a stethoscope, but beware of being misled by your own pulse throbbing in your fingertips. If in any doubt, feel your own pulse at the wrist at the same time as you are trying to feel the patient's.

The oscillometer is sometimes able to record the blood pressure where the sphygmomanometer fails. This instrument detects pulsation in the inflatable cuff. The cuff differs from that used with a sphygmomanometer in that it consists of two cuffs side by side. These are inflated in the usual way and the pressure is recorded by the dial of the oscillometer. Allow the cuff to deflate slowly and as the pressure falls, a point will be reached where the needle of the instrument jerks with every pulse beat. This is the systolic pressure. Take the point where a very definite oscillation occurs and do not be misled by small and indeterminate movements of the needle.

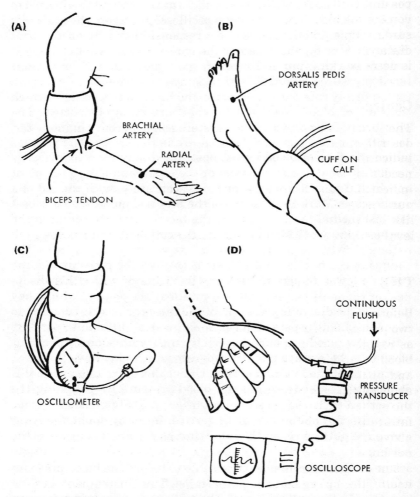

Fig. 5. Methods of measuring blood pressure. (A) Sphygmomanometer cuff on the arm; (B) cuff on the leg; (C) oscillometer; (D) by means of a pressure transducer connected to a cannula in the radial artery.

If it is quite impossible to take the blood pressure in the arms, it may sometimes be taken in the feet. The cuff is placed around the calf. The pulse to be palpated is the dorsalis pedis artery on the dorsum of the foot. It may be felt lying just lateral to the extensor tendon to the big toe. Or you can feel the posterior tibial artery which runs behind the inner ankle bone. Unfortunately it is not possible to take the blood pressure by auscultation at these sites. If you are unable to obtain a pulse in either the arms or the legs make sure that the patient still has a carotid pulse. If he has not, immediately commence the drill for external cardiac compression which is described in Chapter 3.

Central venous pressure

The interpretation of the central venous pressure has been described above. A rise in the central venous pressure usually indicates cardiac failure. Some patients after open heart surgery need a level of venous pressure which might be considered as indicating quite severe heart failure in other patients and the nurse should ask the surgeon responsible at what level he would like the central venous pressure to be maintained and at what level he would consider it to be unacceptably high or low.

THE TREATMENT OF CARDIAC FAILURE

Before resorting to any form of stimulant drug it is essential that two possible causes of cardiac failure are sought for and remedied as rapidly as possible. These are hypoxia and a low circulating blood volume. If the patient is hypoxic, as manifested by cyanosis and either obstructed, laboured or inadequate ventilation with abnormal blood gas values, this must be immediately corrected in the manner to be described in Chapter 4. By the same token heart failure due to a low circulating blood volume, detected as described above, must be treated by blood transfusion or fluid replacement. If neither of these precipitating causes are at fault then it must be assumed that the impaired circulation is due to failure of the pump itself. This may be because the acidity of the blood is abnormal; the heart will deteriorate very rapidly in the presence of metabolic acidosis. Measurement of the blood pH, PCO_2 and standard bicarbonate will indicate whether the patient is suffering from metabolic or respiratory alkalosis or acidosis and will guide the doctor as to the correct treatment to use. It is unlikely that the nurse will have to initiate the treatment of cardiac failure on her own, but she should be aware of the types of drugs which may be used and also some of the undesirable side effects which they may produce.

Digoxin

Digoxin is a purified substance obtained from the foxglove and it exerts its effect in two important ways. It has a direct action on the heart muscle itself and will improve the force with which it contracts; it also depresses the conduction of electrical impulses through the heart. This effect is useful when a patient has an abnormal rapid rhythm of the atria (such as atrial fibrillation or atrial tachycardia) and this rapid rate is conducted to the ventricles which are forced to beat so fast that there is no time available between beats for the heart to fill. When the ventricular rate is too fast cardiac output falls very rapidly. Digoxin prevents the conduction of the impulses from the atria to the ventricles and thus slows the heart. It should not be used to slow the ventricular rate if the tachycardia is due to hypovolaemia.

If an overdose of the drug is given the block in conduction may slow the ventricles or produce coupled beats. Other signs of digoxin toxicity include nausea, frequent extrasystoles or, in extreme cases, ventricular tachycardia or ventricular fibrillation and death. Physicians use varying régimes for the administration of this drug. Digoxin is bound to the heart muscle so that a large initial dose is needed (the digitalizing dose) and this is followed by much smaller doses which are sufficient to replace the drug as it is lost from the body (the maintenance dose). Rapid digitalization may be achieved by giving the drug intravenously, but there are certain risks in doing this. Some physicians prefer to use lanatoside-C (which is derived from the white foxglove) if digitalization by the intravenous route is required, or ouabain which produces a similar effect with great rapidity. Recently methyl digoxin (medigoxin) has been introduced. This is favoured by many doctors for achieving rapid digitalization. The drug may be given more safely by the intramuscular route but will take a little longer to exert its effect. Particular care is needed if the patient is deficient in potassium. If he has been treated with diuretics for many months, potassium will be slowly washed out of the body and this deficiency is accentuated still further if he has recently undergone an operation using a heart-lung machine. The effect of digitalis is exaggerated by a low intracellular potassium concentration and what would be a normal maintenance dose of digoxin for most patients may produce toxic effects after open heart surgery. It is therefore usual to give the drug cautiously in very small increments; as little as 0.0625 mg may produce the desired effect. Potassium should be given in an intravenous drip; we frequently use 40 mmol potassium chloride in a bottle of 500 ml of 5% dextrose infused over 8 hours and on occasions may double the concentration to 80 mmol. If the patient develops frequent extrasystoles on the electrocardiogram he should be given more potassium by drip. Alternatively 1–2 mmol of potassium chloride solution may be given by direct intravenous injection. In other circumstances the administration of potassium by intravenous injection can be dangerous as is explained in Chapter 6. Some centres have found phenytoin sodium, which is more usually employed in the treatment of epilepsy, to be particularly useful in preventing arrhythmias of digitalis intoxication.

Calcium chloride

Calcium ions have a direct stimulating effect on the heart muscle even if there is no measurable deficiency of calcium in the blood. The reason for this is not certain. Calcium may be given either as calcium chloride or calcium gluconate. The latter produces its effect rather more slowly as it has to be metabolized by the liver to release calcium ions. Five ml of the 10% solution given intravenously often produces a remarkable improvement in the function of the heart. Do not forget to warn the patient that he may experience a rather unpleasant warm feeling all over as the drug is being given.

Pressor agents

Three drugs are commonly used to stimulate a flagging heart, adrenaline, dopamine and isoprenaline. I would discount the use of nor-adrenaline which was so popular some years ago. This drug produces its effect by causing intense constriction of the vascular bed without any corresponding stimulating action on the heart itself. Both adrenaline and isoprenaline have two actions on the heart. They may increase the heart rate (chronotropic effect) and they may increase the force of contraction (inotropic effect). There is probably little to choose between them: 2 mg of isoprenaline is dissolved in 500 ml of 5% dextrose and run at a rate necessary to maintain the blood pressure at the required level. This small dose can be remarkably effective. Alternatively, 5 ml of 1:1000 adrenaline is dissolved in 500 ml of the intravenous solution but if elevation of blood pressure can only be obtained by infusing excessive amounts of fluid it may be necessary to double the concentration. Dopamine, and the closely related drug dolbutamine have been introduced recently. They are claimed to increase the cardiac output without stimulating a tachycardia. The kidney blood flow is also increased. These drugs can be combined effectively with adrenaline. A usual dose is 200 mg in 100 ml of 5% dextrose given as a slow infusion. The usual screw clamp or occluder on a drip is not sufficiently sensitive to permit fine control of the drip rate, but screw clips capable of accurate adjustment are obtainable and these should be used if possible. Unfortunately, it will sometimes be found that the blood pressure can only be maintained by using increasingly large doses of the drug. The nurse should chart the number of drops per minute at which the drip is being run so that the doctor will be able to assess whether the heart is improving or failing to respond to his treatment. Drip counters, such as the Ivac machine make controlled infusions much easier to give. A photo-electric cell on the drip chamber senses each drop as it falls and the rate of drip can be maintained at a pre-set level.

The infusion pump can be used to deliver small, continuous doses of a drug over a long period with a greater degree of accuracy than is possible with a screw clip on a drip tube. A syringe containing the drug is connected to an intravenous cannula and clamped in a special stand on which is mounted an electric motor. This motor is used to very slowly depress the plunger of the syringe. Cardiac stimulants, drugs used to treat cardiac dysrhythmias, heparin and the small volumes of intravenous fluids needed in the care of sick babies can all be given in this way.

Drugs used in the treatment of uncontrollable tachycardias

Too rapid a heart rate will quickly lead to a fall in cardiac output. The types of tachycardia which may be produced and their recognition from the electrocardiogram are described in Chapter 5. Although digoxin is indicated to treat many of these, other drugs are used specifically to reduce cardiac irritability. Those most commonly employed are lignocaine, procainamide and propranolol (Inderal). Lignocaine and procainamide are essentially local anaesthetics which when given intravenously reduce the irritability of the heart muscle. Propranolol is one of a group of drugs which produce beta blockade. Stated broadly, the sympathetic nervous system produces its effect on the body through two different types of nerve endings. Beta nerve endings exert their principal effect on the heart itself; the alpha endings vary the degree of constriction or dilatation of the blood vessels. Unfortunately, the heart may be depending upon the drive of the sympathetic nervous system and if this is neutralized by propranolol the blood pressure will fall. The local anaesthetic type of drugs do not have this disadvantage.

Alpha blocking drugs

The condition may be encountered in which the patient is in a low output state with profound constriction of all his peripheral blood vessels and the venous pressure is high. The failing heart is being forced to pump blood against a raised peripheral resistance produced by constriction of the blood vessels. It would, therefore, seem to be advantageous to reduce the work which the heart has to do by reducing the resistance against which it has to pump. This may be achieved by the use of alpha blocking drugs which produce dilation of the blood vessels. Unfortunately, sudden expansion of the vascular bed has the same effect as a sudden massive loss of blood; there is not enough blood available to fill the space created. Hence it will be necessary to transfuse the patient rapidly as the drug is given, using the central venous pressure to guide the rate of the infusion. Another unfortunate side effect is that as the circulation opens up acid waste products are flushed out and the pH of the blood falls. This impairs the contraction of the heart. Therefore, intravenous sodium bicarbonate must be given liberally to counteract the metabolic acidosis. Another reason for using drugs to reduce the peripheral resistance is when it is desirable to lower the blood pressure. The medical treatment of dissecting aneurysm of the aorta depends upon lowering the blood pressure so that the layers of the aortic wall are not split apart. A high blood pressure sometimes occurs after open heart surgery—particularly coronary artery grafting—with an increased risk of bleeding. If sedation with droperidol or chlorpromazine fail to reduce this hypertension, the alpha blockade drug Arfonad (Trimetaphan) or nitroprusside may be used. Because the effects of overdose can be devastating, these powerful drugs are labelled by putting a little methyl blue into the infusion bag. The blue colour should remind you not to flush through the solution rapidly, and to use a drip regulator such as the Ivac. While alpha blocking drugs may be life-saving on occasions, they may also cause rapid death and should not be used without the most careful consideration.

Glucose and insulin

In many patients with a failing circulation, sodium may enter the cells and potassium is forced out. As this process also affects the myocardium, it leads to cardiac failure. The disorder is sometimes called the 'sick cell syndrome'. If the patient is given insulin and glucose, potassium re-enters the cells and sodium is forced out. Experience with this régime is limited but good results have been claimed. This régime is also used to treat acute hyperkalaemia in renal failure (see Chapter 7).

Diuretics

The water and sodium retention of heart failure is treated by drugs which promote increased excretion of urine by the kidney. The pharmacological action of these drugs varies; some counteract the reabsorption of sodium and water by the kidney tubules (frusemide and the mercurial diuretics), some oppose the effect of aldosterone (spironolactone) and others exert an osmotic effect (mannitol). Potassium must be given, in addition, to replace that lost in the ensuing diuresis.

It is important not to give diuretics indiscriminately to correct a low urine output. A low cardiac output, dehydration or tubular necrosis may be the underlying cause, and these must be corrected by the appropriate treatment (see Chapters 3, 6 and 7).

Cortisone

Recent work indicates that in certain types of shock, particularly the variety associated with septicaemia, shunts open up between the arterioles and the veins. Thus, although the cardiac output may be high, blood is short-circuited away from the tissue capillaries. Tissue hypoxia will lead to a metabolic acidosis. The same phenomenon, occurring in the lungs, will interfere with oxygenation of the blood. Large doses of corticosteroids, usually methyl prednisolone, can counteract this shunting most effectively.

CARDIAC TAMPONADE

Cardiac tamponade is the name given to a condition in which the heart is compressed by a collection of blood within the pericardium. This collection compresses the thin-walled atria thereby preventing cardiac filling and this in turn will lead to a fall in cardiac output. Cardiac tamponade may be encountered in patients who have been stabbed in the heart or, more commonly, after cardiac surgery. Even though drainage tubes may be in place within the pericardial cavity and the incision in the pericardium has not been completely closed, it is still possible for blood to accumulate because the tubes have become blocked with clot. Alternatively, the heart may become surrounded with a shell of clot and fresh bleeding may occur within this shell.

Suspect cardiac tamponade in a patient whose blood pressure falls suddenly, especially if quite large quantities of blood have been draining down the tubes and this suddenly ceases. One of the earliest warnings of impending tamponade is that the urine output diminishes. The central venous pressure usually rises unless the patient has a low circulating blood volume. The heart sounds become muffled or inaudible and it may be possible to detect pulsus paradoxus. Normally when a patient inhales the blood pressure falls slightly as blood is pooled in the expanded lung and so less enters the left atrium. This tendency is exaggerated if the patient has cardiac tamponade and the blood pressure may fall by 10 mm of mercury or more during inspiration. Pulsus paradoxus may be detected by taking the blood pressure with a sphygmomanometer cuff. This is inflated to a point where the systolic blood pressure can just be recorded. The patient is then asked to breathe in and the pulse will disappear.

Summon medical help immediately and begin vigorous milking of the drainage tubes; it may be possible to unblock a clotted tube by this method. Under medical direction gentle irrigation of the tubes may succeed in restoring drainage but no time should be lost in preparing the operating theatre so that the chest can be re-opened quickly. Cardiac tamponade is rapidly fatal. On those occasions where the onset of tamponade has been followed almost immediately by cardiac arrest, a few lives have been saved by rapidly opening the chest in the intensive care unit. This not only enables effective internal cardiac massage to be commenced but it also allows the collection of blood in the pericardium to escape.

Chapter 3
The Coronary Care Unit

Myocardial infarction

This term means simply death of myocardium or heart muscle. The condition is a complication of atheromatous disease of the coronary arteries in which fatty deposits are laid down within the inner lining of the arterial walls, with consequent reduction of their lumen. Ulceration and even calcification of these atheromatous plaques may occur. Infarction results when the coronary artery finally becomes occluded, usually as a result of thrombus formation over the atheroma or from a haemorrhage into the plaque resulting in a sudden increase in its size. Occasionally infarction occurs without evidence of coronary occlusion but severe atheromatous disease is always present. In these cases the oxygen requirements of the myocardium have apparently outstripped the ability of the coronary circulation to perfuse the heart for a sufficient period of time to result in death of heart muscle.

Collateral coronary arteries to take over the function of the diseased vessels will develop in response to myocardial ischaemia but the process is slow and takes several years. This may account for the fact that sudden death after myocardial infarction is more common in younger men in whom there has obviously been inadequate time to allow development of collateral vessels.

Myocardial infarction is recognized clinically by a history of severe central chest pain, often gripping or crushing in character, frequently radiating to the neck, jaw and arms. The patient may give a history suggestive of previous angina when the pain was similar, though less severe and related to exercise, emotion or cold weather. He may then have found sublingual glyceryl trinitrate to be of value in relieving his angina but on this occasion the pain does not respond. He is frequently pale, sweaty and apprehensive in appearance.

Electrocardiogram

The electrocardiogram (ECG) reflects the electrical events which precede mechanical contraction of the heart. In the coronary care unit the ECG is usually recorded from an electrode on the chest wall, the waveform displayed upon the patient's oscilloscope depends upon the exact site of the electrode (Fig. 6). The P wave denotes depolarization or electrical stimulation of the atria; this is followed after a short pause (PR interval) by the QRS complex signalling the depolarization of the ventricles, finally the T wave denotes electrical recovery of the heart. This sequence of P wave followed by QRS complex and finally the T wave is always seen in normal (i.e. sinus) rhythm. The ECG is of value not only in the detection of rhythm disturbances but also allows us to confirm the diagnosis of myocardial infarction.

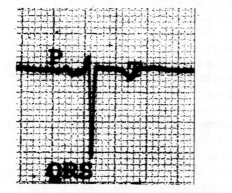 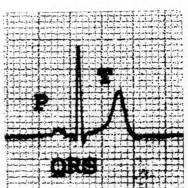

Fig. 6. Normal electrocardiogram. The exact appearance of the ECG varies with the individual lead. The precordial or V leads are often used to monitor arrhythmias. Here are depicted leads V_1 and V_6. Note that although the form of the ECG complexes vary, the P, QRS and T waves are always in the same order.

There is always elevation of the ST segment over the area of infarction and the development of pathological Q waves in the ECG suggests a major degree of myocardial injury. The region of myocardium infarcted may be roughly determined by the distribution of the ST elevation. Changes in leads 1, aVL, V_1 to V_6 suggest infarction in the anterior parts of the ventricles (Fig. 7), leads 2, 3 and aVF reflect events on the inferior or diaphragmatic surface of the heart (Fig. 8).

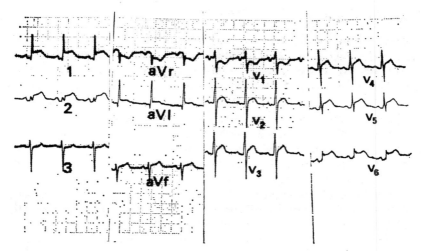

Fig. 7. Anterior infarction. Observe ST elevation in leads 1, 2, aVl, V_4, V_5 and V_6.

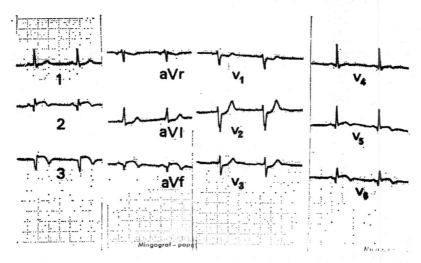

Fig. 8. Inferolateral infarction. ST elevation in leads 2, 3, and aVf, demonstrate the inferior infarction. Similar appearances in leads V_5 and V_6 suggest extension on to the lateral aspects of the ventricle. Pathological Q waves (initial negative deflections) are present in leads 2, 3 and aVf.

Diagnosis is confirmed by detecting a rise in serum enzymes liberated from the injured heart muscle cells. The serum aspartate transaminase (Asp—formerly SGOT) is the enzyme most frequently estimated. Unfortunately it is rather non-specific, being liberated by many tissues other than myocardium, including injured pulmonary tissue. As a result it is elevated in pulmonary infarction and certain abdominal lesions rendering its estimation of little value in the differential diagnosis of acute infarction. An isoenzyme of creatine phosphokinase (MB–CPK) is more specific to injured myocardium and serial estimations of serum CPK levels at 2-hourly intervals allow a quantitative assessment to be made of the extent of the infarction.

Other non-specific signs of inflammation are commonly encountered after myocardial infarction; fever, leucocytosis and elevated ESR. They are of little value in the differential diagnosis of infarction but are of some help in following the progress of the condition.

Coronary care unit

Two major complications await the patient who sustains a myocardial infarction. The extent of muscle injury in the heart may be so severe that the heart fails as a pump and pulmonary oedema or shock result; in spite of the enormous interest in this subject in recent years, there is still relatively little that we can do in this situation. Alternatively, the degree of muscle injury may be relatively slight but an arrhythmia develops which is immediately fatal, as with ventricular fibrillation, or which leads to gross impairment of cardiac function, as in the case of complete heart block or ventricular tachycardia. Coronary care units (CCU) owe their existence to our ability to recognize and treat rhythm disturbances associated with acute infarction.

The design of the CCU in most British hospitals is usually dependent on pre-existing local factors. Ideally there is a need for some cubicle accommodation for the very sick, the noisy, the patient who is being paced and for the most recent admission (the man statistically most likely to cardiac arrest), but some open ward accommodation with the beds arranged in a semi-circle facing the nurse's station is desirable for close contact between nurse and patient and between patients themselves. Although designed with the scientific management of arrhythmias in mind the CCU should have an atmosphere of peace and reassurance for the patient. It is important that our scientific competence does not displace compassion and it is in the maintenance of good morale that the nurse plays a vital role.

General nursing care

The patient's initial need is usually for analgesia. Morphine, so long the traditional powerful analgesic employed in this situation, has two particularly undesirable side effects. Rarely, it provokes hypotension and bradycardia, similar to a simple faint, which responds to elevation of the legs. Although easily treated in the CCU this complication would obviously be more serious in the patient's own home. More frequently morphine causes nausea and vomiting, a most undesirable complication after infarction. Nausea may be diminished by the addition of an antihistamine to the morphine but most units employ diamorphine (5–10 mg parenterally) which is a derivative of morphine but largely free of emetic effects.

There is no ideal posture in which to nurse all patients and it is best to allow them to adopt that which is most comfortable. There are, however, some specific indications for a particular position in bed; a patient with left ventricular failure will always prefer to sit up, whereas hypotension may sometimes be corrected by elevation of the foot of the bed.

Patients are usually kept in the unit for at least 3–4 days. It is our practice to allow patients to feed themselves and to use a bedside commode, although they are washed and shaved by the nursing staff.

It is common clinical procedure to administer oxygen to patients after a heart attack. This is because we know that the pressure of oxygen in the arterial blood (PO_2) is reduced below normal limits and this state of affairs is easily corrected by giving oxygen, providing that the patient is not in shock or pulmonary oedema. A small dead space mask, e.g. an MC mask, should be used. A flow of 4 litres oxygen per minute produces an inspired oxygen concentration of around 40%. There is however no evidence that the routine use of oxygen in this way is of benefit to the patient.

Arrhythmias

Among patients admitted to hospital somewhere between 75 and

90% will experience some form of rhythm disturbance. In the vast majority of cases this will pass unnoticed by the patient and result in no harm, but some will suffer from their arrhythmias. Other rhythm abnormalities, while of no immediate discomfort to the patient, may give warning of serious complications to follow. The CCU nurse must therefore be familiar, not only with the ECG pattern of established arrhythmias but also with their warning signs.

Tachycardias

Supraventricular tachycardias

Sinus tachycardia, i.e. a normal rhythm in excess of 90–100 beats per minute, is almost the rule after infarction and may be of importance in maintaining cardiac output, it may also be an expression of overactivity of the sympathetic component of the autonomic nervous system. Supraventricular tachycardias consist of paroxysmal atrial tachycardia, junctional (nodal) tachycardia, atrial flutter and atrial fibrillation. All result in a sudden increase in heart rate often accompanied by clinical deterioration of the patient. The onset of the arrhythmia may even result in the development of shock or pulmonary oedema.

The commonest supraventricular arrhythmia is atrial fibrillation. The rhythm is recognized by the absence of P waves in the ECG and the totally irregular heart beat. Many of the cardiac contractions will not produce a palpable pulsation at the radial artery and the ventricular rate may only be judged by auscultating the cardiac apex or by observing the ECG on an oscilloscope. The treatment of the patient depends upon the deterioration in his condition. If a state of collapse or pulmonary oedema complicates the onset of atrial fibrillation immediate direct current (d.c.) countershock under general anaesthesia is indicated. The defibrillator must be used in the synchronized phase—the condenser is thereby discharged just after the R or S wave of the QRS complex. Discharge at the time of the T wave may provoke ventricular fibrillation. If the onset of atrial fibrillation results in no serious deterioration in the patient's condition—as judged by the rate of breathing, blood pressure and general appearance—the rhythm should be managed with digoxin. Oral digoxin 0.5 mg at once may be given—the intravenous route may be used if it is felt that intesti-

nal absorption may not be reliable but digoxin must never be given
i.v. if the patient has already been taking the drug. The ventricular rate will not be controlled for some hours by digoxin and short
term slowing of the heart may be achieved by the use of intravenous practolol (10 mg) or verapamil (5–10 mg). These two agents
should not be given together because they may result in asystole.
If, after treatment with digoxin has commenced, the patient
deteriorates d.c.shock may still be used but a low energy discharge
(10–20 joules) reduces the risk of precipitating ventricular fibrillation.

Junctional and atrial tachycardias are less commonly encountered. They produce regular supraventricular tachycardias
(narrow QRS complexes) and their management is similar to
that of atrial fibrillation.

Atrial flutter should always be suspected when the ECG shows a
regular supraventricular tachycardia of 150 per minute. Massage
of the carotid sinus will often slow the ventricular rate temporarily
and reveal the rapid underlying wave form of atrial flutter (Fig. 9).
This rhythm is then treated by digitalization which usually results
in the development of atrial fibrillation although occasionally
reversion to sinus rhythm is achieved.

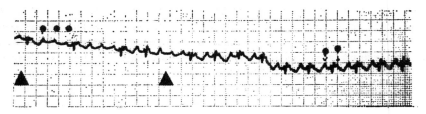

Fig. 9. Atrial flutter. Carotid sinus massage is being applied between
the triangular markers. The rapid flutter waves are easily seen
(dotted). After carotid massage the QRS complexes occur more
frequently and every second flutter wave is lost in the QRS complex.

Although stress has been laid upon the importance of observing
narrow QRS complexes in the diagnosis of supraventricular
arrhythmias it must be stated that occasionally a rapid heart rate
results in functional right bundle branch block (see section on
heart block) and the rhythm then resembles ventricular tachycardia, in its broad QRS complexes. This is because the left branch of
the His bundle recovers its ability to conduct impulses more

rapidly than the right. There is, therefore, a critical rate of impulse from the atrium which will be transmitted by only the left bundle. Often, however, the ventricular rate may be slowed by carotid sinus massage—reduction in rate allows normal conduction to be re-established and with it normal QRS complexes reappear.

All supraventricular tachycardias are frequently preceded by atrial premature beats. In the ECG an atrial premature beat presents as a P wave of differing shape and PR interval from the normal. It may be 'blocked' i.e. fail to repolarize the ventricles or it may occur before electrical recovery of the conduction is completed, and be conducted abnormally through the left branch of the His bundle giving rise to a wide QRS complex which closely resembles a ventricular extrasystole (Fig. 10).

Ventricular tachycardias

Ventricular extrasystoles (VES) or premature beats are extremely common after myocardial infarction and are frequently of little significance. In the past we have regarded complex ventricular ectopic activity—paired ectopics, multifocal or frequent ectopics, short runs of ectopic beats and those extrasystoles interupting the preceding T wave—as warning of impending ventricular fibrillation. Ventricular fibrillation (VF) is often precipitated by a VES (Fig. 11) but the reliability of the so-called warning arrhythmias has been seriously questioned. Nearly half the patients developing VF have no warning arrhythmia and many patients demonstrating complex VES patterns do not develop VF. In an increasing number of CCUs the practice of suppressing ectopic activity with antiarrhythmic drugs like lignocaine has waned but in others such treatment is still practised. The author prefers to concentrate on speedy and effective defibrillation by nurses when VF occurs and to reserve the antiarrhythmic drugs for the management of recurrent VF or ventricular tachycardia. Lignocaine is the agent most frequently used at the present time. Long familiar as a local anaesthetic, this drug has sprung into prominence as a useful antiarrhythmic agent of low toxicity. When administered intravenously in a dose of 100mg an antiarrhythmic effect is rapidly achieved but passes off within less than 20 minutes. Lignocaine may be administered intramuscularly in a dose of approximately 200mg; the effect is then substantially longer. In situations requiring prolonged administration of this drug a con-

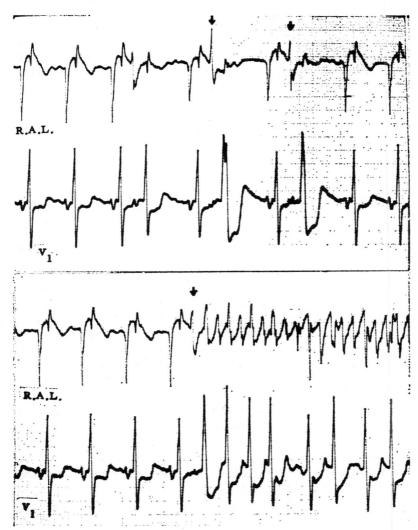

Fig. 10. Atrial premature beats and atrial fibrillations. RAL is recorded from within the right atrium—note how large the P waves appear. You can identify them by matching them up with the more familiar appearances in V_1. In the top illustration the atrial premature beats (arrowed) are conducted to the ventricles abnormally and produce broad QRS complexes resembling ventricular premature beats. In the lower illustration the atrial premature beat precipitates an episode of atrial fibrillation. Note the total irregularity of the QRS complexes in V_1.

stant intravenous infusion is used at a dose level of 1–4 mg/min. Close observation is required to prevent overdosage and the toxic effects of the drug. The elderly patient and those with hepatic disorders are particularly liable to develop such unwanted effects. Confusion, hallucinations and coma have been reported from excessive lignocaine, myocardial depression with cardiac failure may occur as well as impaired atrioventricular conduction. Prevention of these effects is better than detection since the blood level of lignocaine may take more than 2 hours to fall after discontinuing a prolonged infusion.

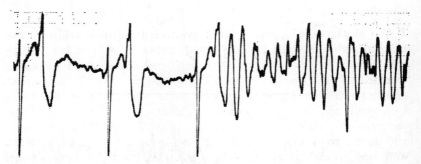

Fig. 11. Ventricular premature beats (extrasystoles) falling on the T wave of a preceding QRS complex. The third premature beat appears to provoke the onset of ventricular fibrillation.

Alternative or supplementary antiarrhythmic drugs are procainamide, mexiletine and disopyramide. It must be remembered that they all depress the pumping power of the cardiac musculature and may provoke heart failure.

Ventricular tachycardia consists of a rapid sequence of ventricular extrasystoles without intervening sinus beats. It frequently proceeds to the development of ventricular fibrillation but it may persist unchanged for several hours. It is recognized by its rapid rate and broad complexes but may be simulated by a supraventricular tachycardia with aberrant atrioventricular conduction as discussed above. There is always clinical deterioration of the patient and an immediate intravenous injection of lignocaine or procainamide should be given. If this fails to produce a return to sinus rhythm the patient should be anaesthetized and normal rhythm restored by d.c. counter shock.

Ventricular fibrillation is the classic 'cardiac arrest' and must explain many cases of sudden death from myocardial infarction before admission to hospital can be achieved. A useless diffuse quivering of cardiac muscle results. Ventricular extrasystoles may herald the onset of ventricular fibrillation, but it often occurs without warning.

Cardiac arrest due to ventricular fibrillation in a CCU should be treated by immediate defibrillation, but where this is impossible the circulation and respiration must be sustained by cardiac massage and ventilation until defibrillation can be achieved.

Cardiac arrest—resuscitation

If the electrocardiograph reveals ventricular fibrillation or the carotid pulse is impalpable, do not waste time in debate as to whether the heart sounds can be heard, commence cardiac massage immediately. External cardiac massage requires a firm base against which to support the spine during sternal compression and CCU beds are usually equipped with fracture boards and thin, compressible mattresses. The nurse places herself at the patient's right side, the heel of one hand on the lower third of the sternum and the heel of the other hand on top of it. Firm, regular depression of the sternum to a distance of 3–5 cm at a rate of 60–70 per minute is then commenced. Keep the arms rigid and use the weight of your trunk to provide the compressing force (Fig. 12).

Failure to place the hands correctly can result in serious complications. If pressure is applied too low the xiphisternal process may be fractured and driven into the liver. Pressure applied lateral to the sternum may fracture a rib, driving the broken bone into the lung or heart. Fatigue is a commoner cause of bad massage than ignorance and few people can maintain effective massage for more than a few minutes, particularly with the patient on a bed and the operator standing. The efficiency of massage may be checked by palpating the femoral pulses which should be easily felt when massage is adequate. Palpation of the carotid pulse can be difficult in a patient who is being jerked by cardiac compression.

Ventilation is commenced by extending the patient's neck fully to ensure that the airway is patent. Initially artificial respiration is started by the mouth to mouth method. The patient's nostrils are gently pinched together with the left hand and the lungs inflated by blowing directly into the patient's open mouth. The effectiveness of ventilation can be easily checked by ensuring that the

patient's chest is expanding during the operation. This technique
is quickly replaced by the insertion of an oropharyngeal airway
and ventilation with a self-inflating (AMBU) bag. The Brooke
airway is another useful first aid device but truly efficient artificial ventilation may only be achieved after endotracheal intubation. It is important to coordinate the efforts at ventilation
and cardiac massage, say one ventilation every sixth external
massage.

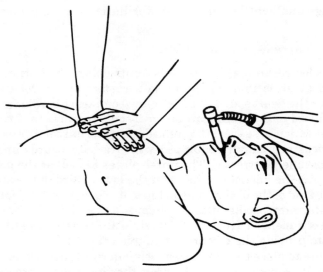

Fig. 12. External cardiac massage.

An attempt must be made to defibrillate the heart at the earliest
opportunity; delay rapidly reduces the chances of successful cardioversion. The defibrillator is charged to 300 joules and the switch
or indicator set to the 'manual' position because the ECG contains
no regular wave form to trigger the 'synchronized' discharge.

The electrode paddles are covered with an electrolyte jelly and
pressed firmly against the chest wall, one over the apex and one to
the right of the sternum. Many paddles are spring loaded and firm
pressure is necessary to ensure good contact within the paddle. An
added safety measure is for two operators to hold one paddle each,
having first wiped their hands free of any electrode jelly, saline or
perspiration. Once the condensor is charged and the paddles in
place it must be checked that no one is in contact with the patient,

after which the condensor is discharged by pressing either the switch on the machine or the button on the electrode handle. The discharge of current should make the patient jerk. If sparking between the paddles and the patient occurs, contact is imperfect and severe burns may be produced (Fig. 13).

An acidosis develops rapidly as a result of impaired tissue perfusion and inefficient ventilation. This must be corrected, both in order to facilitate cardioversion and to prevent the cardiac depressant effects of the acidosis. Sodium bicarbonate (8.4%) 1 mmol/ml is infused usually to a dose of 100–400 mmol depending on the duration of arrest.

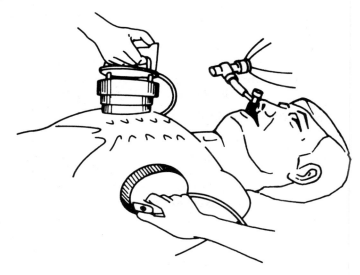

Fig. 13. External defibrillation.

Failure to convert from ventricular fibrillation to sinus rhythm may be due to inadequate correction of the severe acidosis and this can be rapidly checked by estimating the pH of arterial blood. If there has been considerable delay before defibrillation is attempted the fibrillation waves on the ECG become very fine and electrical conversion is then more difficult. It is worthwhile under these circumstances coarsening the wave formation with adrenaline or isoprenaline to facilitate defibrillation.

After successful resuscitation it is customary to administer antiarrhythmic drugs to prevent recurrence of the ventricular fibrillation. Finally, the patient's ability to ventilate adequately must be checked because a short period of assisted ventilation may be required after resuscitation. In the event of severe damage to the bony cage of the thorax resulting from cardiac massage the condition of flail chest may result, demanding a prolonged period of mechanical ventilation (see Chapter 4).

Bradycardias

Sinus or nodal bradycardia are very common after inferior infarction. When the rate falls to around 50 per minute the patient may become hypotensive and develop ventricular arrhythmias. Most bradycardias of this type are easily corrected by administration of atropine 0.3 mg intravenously, a low dose which may be repeated within a few minutes if there is no increase in heart rate. Rarely the bradycardia is resistant to atropine and pacing from the atrium may be required.

Heart block (atrioventricular block)

The bundle of His travels in the posterior part of the interventricular septum, AV block is therefore relatively common in posterior or inferior infarction. First degree AV block consists of a lengthening of the PR interval to more than 0.2 seconds and results in no disability to the patient. Second degree block consists of two main patterns, the Wenckebach phenomenon (Fig. 14) in which there is

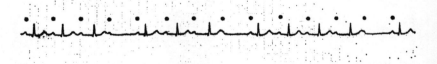

Fig. 14. Wenckebach phenomenon. All the P waves are marked. Note that the distance between the P wave and QRS complex (PR interval) gradually increases until the 4th P wave is not conducted at all. The cycle is repeated.

a gradual increase in PR interval until a 'dropped' beat eventually occurs and the Mobitz type II pattern in which the PR interval is constant but occasionally a P wave is not conducted to the ventricles and again a 'dropped' beat occurs. Although both patterns are called second degree block their significance is very different. Wenckebach phenomenon is common in inferior infarctions and may precede the development of complete block in which the ventricular pacemaker is relatively fast and of normal QRS configuration (Fig. 15). Mobitz block, on the other hand, is commonly seen

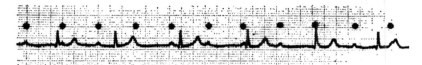

Fig. 15. Complete heart block in inferior infarction. There is no constant relationship between the P waves (dotted) and the QRS complexes. Note that the QRS complexes are fairly regular, of normal appearance and occur at a rate of between 50 and 60 per minute.

after anterior infarction and leads to a form of complete block characterized by a slow ventricular rate often associated with the emergence of ventricular ectopic beats or the development of heart failure or shock (Fig. 16).

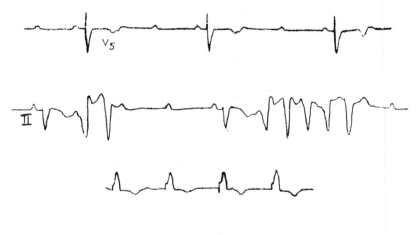

PACED

Fig. 16. Complete heart block. Anterior infarction. As in Fig. 8, there is no fixed relationship between P and QRS complexes but here the QRS complexes have a much slower rate and are broad and notched in appearance. In the middle tracing frequent ventricular premature beats occur. The third tracing shows the ECG during cardiac pacing. The rhythm is now regular and of an adequate rate.

Another pattern associated with the development of complete block after anterior infarction is the combination of right bundle branch block and left axis or right deviation (Fig. 17).

Complete atrioventricular block means that the ventricles must beat at their own inherent rhythm. The ventricular rate may, after inferior infarction, be as fast as 50–56 per minute and require no therapy. After anterior infarction, however, it is usually much slower and does not permit an adequate cardiac output and serious ventricular arrhythmias are likely to develop.

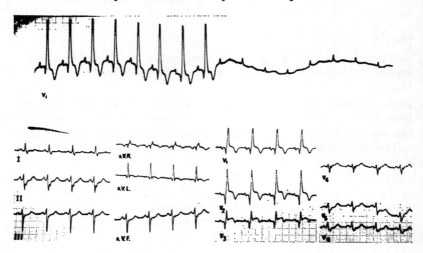

Fig. 17. Anterior infarction with right bundle branch block and left axis deviation. The V₁ rhythm strip shows the onset of ventricular asystole.

Complete block may be treated by drugs which increase the frequency of ventricular pacemaker discharge or by direct stimulation of the heart via an electrode pacemaker situated within the right ventricle. Infusion of suitable drugs, e.g. isoprenaline, may be difficult to control over three or four days and most units prefer the technique of transvenous pacemaking. A unipolar or bipolar pacing catheter is introduced percutaneously into a subclavian vein and advanced under fluoroscopic control to the apex of the right ventricle. Some CCUs prefer to insert the catheter into a jugular vein and others use the antecubital or even the femoral veins.

Stimulus is provided from an external pacemaker which produces regular pulses of electric current. Complete block is practically always transient after infarction and in survivors normal conduction usually returns in two to four days. There may be competition between normally conducted beats and the artificial pacemaker which can be hazardous and result in ventricular fibrillation. A demand pacemaker is used which ensures delivery of a stimulus only if the ventricle fails to beat spontaneously. The true value of pacing in complete block following infarction is difficult to assess but one estimate suggests that the mortality of this complication has been reduced from around 70% to approximately 40% by the introduction of demand pacing.

When the pacing catheter is first inserted it should be possible to pace with a stimulus of 1 volt or less. The voltage may need to be increased after the first few hours of pacing but a sudden and marked increase in the voltage required to pace the heart suggests that the tip of the catheter has been displaced and may even have punctured the myocardium. The true state of affairs may be established and rectified by radiological screening and replacement of the electrode.

The electrode may conduct an unwanted stimulus to the heart, e.g. a nurse touching an oscilloscope which holds a static electrical charge who simultaneously comes into contact with the terminal of the catheter electrodes will allow the static charge to be transmitted to the ventricle with possibly disastrous results. All terminals from the electrodes should therefore be well insulated.

Cardiac failure

Acute myocardial infarction tends to involve mainly the left ventricle and if the myocardial injury is sufficiently severe pulmonary oedema may result. The patient is severely dyspnoeic, is most comfortable when propped up or sitting forward and coughs frothy, frequently blood stained sputum. The coarse rattling of oedematous fluid within the lungs is usually audible without the need of a stethoscope.

Diamorphine will make the patient feel less dyspnoeic and the pulmonary oedema is reduced by propping the patient upright and administering a diuretic. A powerful diuretic with prompt action is intravenous frusemide (40 mg) or bumetanide 1 mg. Frusemide is the most widely used diuretic in acute pulmonary oedema and the drug may be continued by the intramuscular or oral route. The use of these powerful diuretics on more than two or three occasions results in severe potassium loss and an oral potassium chloride preparation must be prescribed.

The mechanical performance of the heart is improved by digitalis and again it is usual to initiate digitalization in emergencies by the intravenous route. Finally a high concentration of oxygen is usually given to the patient by means of a small volume dead space mask with a high oxygen flow setting.

Rarely pulmonary oedema is sufficiently severe to warrant treatment with venous tourniquets on the limbs or even venesection, but the advent of the newer diuretics has made these procedures rare.

Shock

Confusion exists over the very meaning of this term. The pain and fear of infarction alone may provoke a picture of pallor, grey skin and sweating. In this country, however, we tend to reserve the term 'shock' for patients in whom there persists a picture of hypotension (systolic pressure less than 80 mmHg), oliguria, mental confusion and poor peripheral blood flow, even after adequate analgesia, elevation of the feet and administration of oxygen. There is frequently an acidosis and a degree of hypoxaemia which is not corrected by conventional oxygen therapy.

The prognosis is very poor and as witness to this there is a long list of suggested treatments—pressor agents, steroids, hyperbaric oxygen, sometimes plasma expansion, mechanical support of the circulation and emergency surgical revascularization. At this time there is no reliable form of therapy for this state and we must note that the degree of myocardial injury found at autopsy among this group is considerable. Although the search for an effective treatment must be continued it may be that these patients represent the hard core of patients whose death is almost inevitable. Research is currently being conducted into the limitation of infarct size or the protection of the myocardium in an attempt to reduce the incidence of shock.

Other complications

Pericarditis

This is common and often responsible for recurrence and persistence of central chest pain. A friction rub is often audible, although frequently transient. No specific therapy other than analgesia and reassurance is required.

Ventricular rupture

Rupture of the ventricular wall, although typically a late complication at 2 or 3 weeks after infarction, is occasionally encountered in the first few days. Alternatively, the ventricular septum may rupture and the torrential shunting of blood thus produced may lead to cardiac failure.

Arterial embolism

Emboli may arise from thrombus situated in the left ventricular wall over the area of infarction and may be carried to the limbs, brain, kidneys or mesentery. The onset of sudden pain in a limb accompanied by loss of pulses, coldness and pallor should suggest embolism. Occasionally the dramatic picture is seen of a massive clot lodging in the aortic bifurcation—the so-called saddle embolus. There is severe pain in the lower back with total obliteration of the circulation distal to this point. Embolectomy is often required urgently in cases of peripheral embolism.

Pulmonary embolus

This is a late complication rarely seen during the patient's short stay in a CCU. When encountered it is usually in the patient who has been heavily sedated, possibly after multiple episodes of cardiac arrest, or in the patient who is very elderly or suffering from protracted cardiac failure.

Chapter 4
Maintaining Adequate Respiration

In its strict, physiological sense, respiration is the term used to describe the uptake of oxygen and elimination of carbon dioxide by the cell. Here it will be used in its more familiar meaning, as the function of the lung. Respiration is obviously of overriding importance to the nurse concerned with the management of patients with lung disease or the post-operative care of thoracic surgical procedures. However, the care of the lungs must be a major consideration in any seriously ill patient.

Death from pulmonary causes is common in those suffering from major injuries, from unconsciousness or chronic illness necessitating prolonged recumbency. The pulmonary complications of abdominal surgery are well known and must be watched for with unceasing vigilance. As with most other aspects of intensive care, prevention of trouble is even more important than the treatment of established disease.

In order to understand the common sense and practical measures to be described, it is first necessary to appreciate something of the physiology of the lung. The lung enables the blood to pick up oxygen from the air and to eliminate carbon dioxide. Its structure is devised to bring blood and air into intimate contact. It follows that the two important components of lung function are ventilation, that is, the mechanism whereby gases are moved in and out of the lung, and the pulmonary circulation. Pulmonary disease interferes with either one or both of these components, with the result that the oxygen saturation of the blood will be reduced (hypoxia) and the carbon dioxide content will be elevated (hypercapnia). The effects are far-reaching and may be catastrophic. The brain withstands hypoxia poorly, and severe oxygen depletion will lead to heart failure. As the heart and lungs function as one unit, heart failure may well lead to pulmonary oedema which in turn impairs oxygenation of the blood. The vicious circle thus initiated will kill

60

the patient unless desperate and dramatic measures are successful. How much better it is to prevent pulmonary disease, or, if this is not possible, to recognize the signs of impending trouble early and to treat them promptly, than to be forced to apply heroic measures later.

To enable the lungs to effect the exchange of gases, certain conditions must be fulfilled.

1. There must be a clear air passage between the lips and alveoli.
2. The lungs must be expanded so that they fill the pleural cavities.
3. The chest wall and the diaphragm must move in and out to exert their bellows effect on the lung.
4. The substance of the lung (the parenchyma) must be free from disease.

Each of these will be considered in more detail.

MAINTENANCE OF THE AIRWAY

If an unconscious patient is allowed to lie on his back, his tongue may fall backwards and obstruct the upper air passages. It follows that such patients should be nursed on their sides. If respiratory obstruction of this type is encountered it may speedily be corrected by lifting the jaw forwards with firm pressure behind its angles. As the tongue is attached to the jaw it will be drawn away from the back wall of the throat. An anaesthetic airway may be inserted. The trick for inserting an airway is to put it into the mouth with its tip against the palate (i.e. upside-down). Once it has been introduced fully it is twisted through 180°. If this method is not adopted the tip of the airway will catch under the tongue.

Acute obstruction of the air passages by inhaled foreign bodies or vomit is a dramatic emergency, easily recognized. The treatment is obvious. The obstruction must be removed as quickly as possible. This usually requires the help of a doctor, but the nurse should waste no time in bringing the trolley with laryngoscopes, a bronchoscope, long bronchoscopy forceps and suction equipment to the bedside. Ideally, bronchoscopy should be performed under anaesthesia (general or local) in an operating theatre, but in extreme emergency it may be necessary to perform bronchoscopy in the bed. For this reason, the bronchoscopy trolley should be ready to use at any time in the ICU.

Less obvious, but far more common, is obstruction of the air passages by bronchial secretions. The bronchi are coated with a thin layer of mucus. This traps fine particles of dust and dirt which have been inhaled. The respiratory mucous membrane is provided with myriads of fine cilia which propel the mucus towards the trachea. If a sufficiently large blob of mucus collects at the sensitive lower end of the trachea, it provokes the desire to cough. If the patient has chronic bronchitis or is a heavy smoker, mucus is produced in excessive quantities. Both of these conditions impair the ciliary action, indeed, heavy smoking transforms the lining of the trachea to a structure which resembles skin and has patches without cilia. Unless secretions can be eliminated by coughing they will accumulate, obstruct the bronchi and eventually 'drown' the patient.

When a bronchus is obstructed, the oxygen in the part of the lung beyond the block is absorbed and the lung collapses (atelectasis). As secretions collect and obstruct further bronchi, segments, then lobes, and eventually the whole lung will become atelectatic. The clinical presentation of atelectasis may be acute or insidious in onset. Suspicion should be aroused if the patient becomes breathless, with a rising pulse rate and a cyanotic tinge. The latter sign is transitory and may disappear after an hour or two as the circulation to the affected section of lung shuts down and the shunting of desaturated blood from the right to the left side of the heart ceases. Clinical examination and a radiograph of the chest will confirm the diagnosis. It will be seen that the ability to cough effectively is all-important in keeping the airways clear. It is useful to understand the mechanism of coughing. The lungs are first filled with air by a deep inspiration, then the glottis is closed. Forced expiration against the closed glottis builds up high pressures in the airways, so that when the glottis opens, air is expelled at a speed approaching 200 m.p.h., carrying sputum with it like the cork from a popgun. With this picture in mind, it is not difficult to list the sort of conditions which will impede coughing. Violent movement of the chest wall is difficult if the patient is elderly, comatose or unconscious. The pain of fractured ribs or a recent surgical incision in the chest wall or upper abdomen likewise inhibit coughing. Mechanical interference with chest wall movement because of paralysis of the diaphragm or because the rigidity of the thorax has been impaired by multiple fractures or surgical excision also plays a part. Finally, inability to close the glottis because of paralysis of the recurrent laryngeal nerve produced by lung or thyroid excision, or because the patient has a tracheostomy or endotracheal tube in place, may also lead to retention of sputum and atelectasis (Fig. 18).

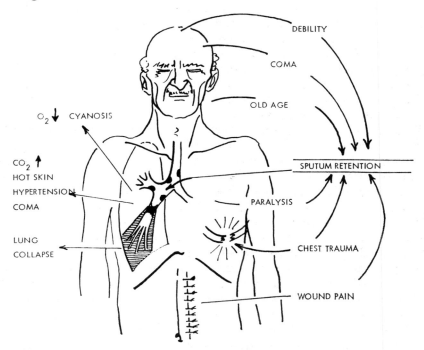

Fig. 18. The factors leading to sputum retention.

NURSING CARE OF THE AIRWAYS

Prevention of sputum retention

The object of nursing care of the airways is to prevent atelectasis. From what has already been said it will be obvious that deep breathing and coughing must be encouraged, and the responsibility for this falls as heavily on the nursing staff who are with the patient throughout the day as it does on the physiotherapist. The sitting position is best for deep breathing and coughing unless contra-indicated by hypotension, unconsciousness or spinal injury. It is common experience that one always sits up in bed if troubled by a bad bout of coughing at night. If the patient has to lie flat then he must be turned frequently from side to side. This is to encourage secretions to drain under gravity from each lung in turn. Babies may need to be turned as often as every 15 minutes.

The nurse must learn to recognize the distinctive bubbling respiration of a patient who is developing sputum retention, and having recognized it, spare no effort to ensure a clear airway. Neglect this duty, and the inevitable result will be death by drowning. A cheerful, reassuring air is important. Patients are often afraid to cough after surgery, partly because of pain and partly because they fear that they may rupture their wounds. Sometimes they seem to have forgotten how to cough and can only manage noisy forced expiration. If the patient is hypoxic, or drowsy from carbon dioxide retention, he will often be uncooperative and 'difficult'. Patience and firmness will be needed if such patients are to be encouraged to clear their airways without the need for bronchoscopy. Stand to one side of the patient, supporting the wound, if one is present, with two hands. Alternatively, the patient can support his own wound, either with his hands or a broad webbing strap wrapped round his chest. Such straps are commercially available and have the additional refinement of a Velcro pad which holds the two ends of the strap together. Tell him to take three deep breaths and to cough after the third. Often, the 'tickle' produced by deep breathing will provoke a cough. If the patient's efforts are weak, firmly compress his chest with your hands as he coughs. This additional help may succeed in expelling sputum.

A pressure-cycled ventilator such as the Bird can be used with a mouthpiece. The patient wears a noseclip, holds the mouthpiece between the lips and inhales. With the machine on the 'trigger' setting this causes a puff of gas to be delivered which supplements the patient's own efforts and inflates his chest. A patient on the verge of respiratory failure can often be spared the ordeal of endotracheal intubation and mechanical ventilation by this technique and it is helpful in assisting with coughing and the expectoration of sputum. Of course he must be conscious and cooperative, and it may need patience to teach him how to use the machine. Try it yourself to get an insight into the problems. Once they have mastered the trick some patients are happy to give themselves 'puff therapy' without supervision.

Pain is the commonest reason for difficulty in coughing—and here the nurse will face a dilemma. The most effective analgesic drugs, such as morphia and omnopon are also respiratory depressants. This effect is particularly noticeable if the drugs are given in large doses at infrequent intervals—the familiar 20 mg of omnopon every 6 hours. This mode of administration ensures that the patient is too heavily drugged to cough at the beginning of the 6-hour period; after about 3 or 4 hours the pain will be sufficiently severe to suppress coughing until the next dose is due, and the cycle is repeated. It is surely more logical to use smaller doses of the drug, and to give them more frequently, thereby assuring a steady level of analgesia which is enough to dull the pain without making the patient so drowsy that he cannot cooperate. 10–15 mg of omnopon every 3–4 hours usually achieves this. The appropriate dose must be judged from the patient's size and his response to the drug.

Sputum retention is also more likely to occur if the secretions are sticky and tenacious, and this is more likely if the patient is dehydrated—another example of disorders in one system producing troubles in another. Most of the drugs which have been devised to help coughing (the expectorants) are ineffective. By far the best aid for the patient with difficulty in coughing is a hot drink, such as tea. Some assistance may be had from steam inhalations or the well-known tinct. benz. co. or menthol. Success is claimed for the drug, n-acetyl cysteine, which thins tenacious secretions. It appears to do this by stimulating the bronchial glands to produce water mucus. Alevaire (Winthrop Labs., Surbiton, Surrey) can be used in a nebulizer and is also effective in thinning sticky secretions.

Finally, the role of cough suppressant drugs must be considered. There is no place for these if there is sputum in the air passages, but an irritating, tickling cough which does not produce sputum but keeps the patient awake, may be relieved by the familiar linctuses, such as Gee's and linctus codeine, or the more powerful drugs codeine and physeptone.

Bronchospasm

The walls of the smaller bronchi contain smooth muscle which can contract, and thereby narrow the lumen of the air passages. This is the mechanism underlying the wheezing of asthma. The interference with the easy passage of gases in and out of the lung can cause distressing breathlessness. A stethoscope on the chest detects musical whistling noises with every breath. There are many drugs which are effective in relieving bronchospasm, of which the most important are adrenaline, isoprenaline, ephedrine, salbutamol, disodium cromoglycate (Intal, Johannesburg), and methoxyphenamine.

Management of sputum retention

Inevitably, some patients will develop pulmonary collapse from retained secretions despite the most assiduous care. The warning signs have been described above. Sometimes a short application of intensive physiotherapy will succeed in dislodging the sputum, but the chances of success once atelectasis has become established are not great. The absorption of gases from beyond the block means that the popgun effect of coughing will be lost. Sputum can no longer be blown out; it is just possible that it can be shaken or drained out. It is obviously pointless, and rather inhumane, to continue to harry a patient who has a collapsed lobe despite his prolonged efforts in the face of pain and weakness. If he cannot get rid of his sputum, his medical and nursing attendants must do it for him. The progression of methods to be adopted is as follows:

Nasotracheal aspiration

A suction catheter passed through the mouth seldom does more than aspirate secretions in the pharynx, and perhaps initiate a fit of coughing by irritating the glottis. It is unusual for the catheter to pass on into the trachea. A more certain technique is nasotracheal aspiration, which is particularly useful if the patient can manage to cough sputum as far as the trachea, but cannot muster the energy to expel it any further. The bubbling, gargling type of breathing is characteristic. The patient is propped up in bed. The tongue is grasped with a gauze swab and pulled forward as a lubricated catheter is passed through the nose into the pharynx. The tip should now be directly over the vocal cords. As the patient inhales the catheter is rapidly threaded through the nose and on into the trachea. Success will be signalled by the bout of coughing this provokes. Although the experience is not very pleasant for the patient, and firmness and confidence is needed on the part of the attendant, the clearing of the airway thus obtained is very gratifying and may avoid the need for more elaborate procedures (Fig. 19). We have, on occasions, left the suction catheter lying in the trachea, where it may be used to aspirate secretions for some days without causing erosion of the vocal cords.

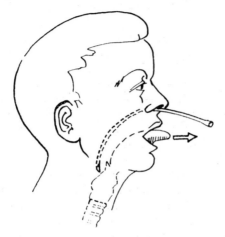

Fig. 19. Nasotracheal aspiration. The tongue is pulled forward as the catheter is threaded through the nose.

Bronchoscopy

Established atelectasis, or the failure of the simpler methods described above indicate the need for bronchoscopy. Although the nurse will not be required to do this, she should be able to set up a bronchoscopy trolley and know how to assist. It is desirable that bronchoscopy sets should be available in sterile packs, ready for immediate use, and be in working order. The lead is attached to a battery box or other appropriate power source. If the light fails to come on, first check that the bulb is not blackened, and then check the electrical connections. Bulbs and leads are vulnerable and need frequent replacement. Be careful to turn up the power supply slowly—a surge of current will fuse the bulb. The modern cold light instruments are more robust and reliable. The bronchoscope should be smeared with lubricant. Two suction cannulae should be available—make sure that the gum elastic tips are securely screwed on, or they will become detached and lost in the bronchial tree (Fig. 20).

The patient is most conveniently bronchoscoped lying flat; urgent bronchoscopy in a standard hospital bed may be performed with the patient propped up and the operator standing on a box, working over the bed head. Anaesthesia will not be necessary under conditions of extreme urgency, or in the unconscious subject. For more elective procedures general anaesthesia is popular in many centres, and certainly provides excellent working conditions, but if local anaesthesia is to be used, a nebulizer spray, a pair of Krause's forceps, gauze pledgets, a 2-ml syringe and fine needle and a bottle of 4% lignocaine or cocaine solution must be provided.

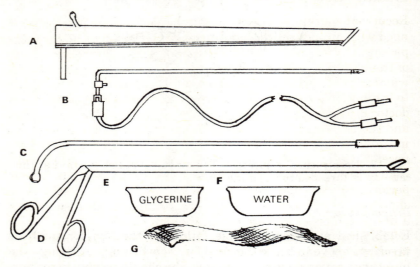

Fig. 20. Equipment required for bronchoscopy. (A) Bronchoscope; (B) light carrier, bulb and flex; (C) metal suction tube with gum elastic tip; (D) biopsy or grasping forceps; (E) glycerine for lubrication; (F) water; (G) gauze swab.

The mouth and pharynx are sprayed, a little local anaesthetic is injected directly into the trachea and pledgets of gauze, soaked in the solution, are grasped in the Krause forceps and passed over the tongue to anaesthetize the superior laryngeal nerve. The surgeon should be provided with a gauze swab to protect the patient's lips and teeth. The assistant inserts the sucker tip into the broncho-scope as it is inconvenient for the surgeon to repeatedly lift his head away from the instrument every time he needs to pass a sucker. If local anaesthesia has been used, the patient must be starved for about 4 hours afterwards as food and drink will pass into the trachea without the patient's knowledge.

The modern flexible fibreoptic bronchoscope not only extends the range of the surgeons vision out to the smaller branches of the bronchial tree, but it can also be passed down the lumen of an indwelling endotracheal tube. Each bronchus can be conveniently sucked out under direct vision without extubating the patient. The technique is remarkably effective and simple.

Tracheal intubation

Recurrent sputum retention, despite bronchoscopy, may be managed with an indwelling endotracheal tube for up to 10 days. The passage of these tubes, and their subsequent management, is one of the basic techniques in intensive care, with an application far wider than the aspiration of secretions (see Chapter 5). The ability to intubate the trachea should be part of the stock-in-trade of any doctor concerned with intensive care. A clear airway is assured, and the lungs can be inflated with an Ambu bag, an anaesthetic machine or ventilator. Endotracheal intubation is an immediate necessity in the treatment of cardiac arrest and major chest injuries. While it is not expected that the nurse should be able to perform this, it would be very worthwhile to ask an anaesthetist to show you the basic steps. The knowledge might enable you to save a life if medical help were not available.

The first essential is to obtain a view of the vocal cords with a laryngoscope. Most laryngoscopes are designed for use by a right-handed person, and have a flange running down the right-hand edge of the blade. Grasp the instrument with your left hand, and stand at the head of the patient. Insert the blade into the mouth so that the flange holds the tongue towards the patient's left. As you pass the blade over the back of the tongue, lift, and the epiglottis will come into your view as a little flap. Guide the beak of the blade into the space between the epiglottis and the front wall of the throat, and lift the whole of the larynx firmly towards the ceiling. The vocal cords will now be seen—they are two pale pink bands with the dark entry into the trachea between them. Pick up a lubricated endotracheal tube with your right hand and pass it into the trachea. Inflate the cuff and attach the tube to an Ambu or anaesthetic bag. Give the bag one or two trial squeezes to ensure that the chest rises and falls. Even the most experienced operators have mistakenly intubated the oesophagus on occasions. The bag should be compressed rhythmically and with enough force to inflate the chest visibly. Adjust the gas flows to a level where the bag refills after each breath. About 6 l/min is usually sufficient.

A word of caution about the management of inflatable cuffs on endotracheal and tracheostomy tubes. Over-inflation of these cuffs will cause ischaemic necrosis of the cartilaginous rings of the trachea which will lead to stricture formation. The management of a tracheal stricture is one of the most difficult problems encountered in surgery. Therefore the cuff should be inflated until it just produces an airtight fit, and no more. This point may be gauged by listening to breath sounds. Squeeze the bag with the cuff deflated and notice the snoring sound produced by air escaping alongside the tube and through the vocal cords. Now slowly inflate the cuff and notice the volume of air which has been injected at the point where this snoring noise ceases. This volume should never be exceeded. It is the practice in some centres to deflate the cuff for a short period every hour in order to minimize pressure effects. Such modifications as an alternately inflated double cuff system or soft, floppy cuffs are claimed to reduce this hazard. The special problems of tracheal intubation in children are described in Chapter 9. Before the endotracheal tube is removed the patient is carefully watched during a trial period in which he breathes on his own without ventilator support. The chest wall movements must be adequate, the skin and nail beds must remain pink and blood gas estimates performed immediately after disconnecting the ventilator and an hour later must be within normal limits. It is usual practice to attach an extension to the endotracheal tube which increases the patient's 'dead space'. This prevents him from blowing off too much carbon dioxide. If all is well, the trachea is sucked out and the tube is removed.

Tracheostomy

Tracheostomy was an operation performed with great frequency a few years ago, but now that endotracheal tubes made of non-irritant plastics have been developed the indications have become more limited. These may be briefly stated as the necessity for mechanical ventilation or aspiration of secretions for longer than 10 days, following excision of the larynx and upper respiratory tract obstruction. Such classical indications as diphtheria are seldom encountered these days. There is some variation of opinion as to the length of time which an endotracheal tube should be left in place before performing tracheostomy. The principal complications of prolonged intubation is pressure necrosis of the vocal cords. If it is obvious that the patient is going to need to be ventilated for 2 or 3 weeks we proceed to tracheostomy at 5 days, but if his condition is improving, we would extend this period to a week in the hope that tracheostomy can be avoided. Some units leave endotracheal tubes in place for 2 or 3 weeks and do not appear to have problems.

The practical details of the operation need not concern the nurse, but she should be aware of the various patterns of openings in the trachea. Some surgeons prefer a simple slit or circular hole; many favour the Björk operation in which a trapdoor flap is cut and turned forward to be sutured to the inferior lip of the skin incision (Fig. 21). This flap provides a useful guide when the tracheostomy tube is changed. The value of a tube in the trachea which can be tolerated for many weeks is obvious. It provides a means for clearing the airway of obstructing secretions or a port to which a mechanical ventilator can be connected. However, there are serious disadvantages which particularly concern the nurse. Properly managed, tracheostomy is a life-saving operation. Inefficient nursing will inevitably lead to complications which will frequently cause death. Once tracheostomy has been performed, the patient will be unable to cough effectively, because the glottis is above the tube. Hence he is totally dependent upon the nurse for the removal of sputum from his bronchial tree. Furthermore, he is deprived of the humidifying action of the nose and upper air passages. If dry air enters the trachea, the secretions become sticky and difficult to

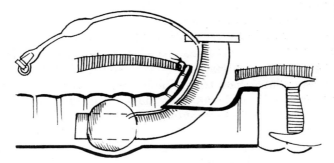

Fig. 21. Flap tracheostomy with cuffed tracheostomy tube in position.

aspirate and eventually will form crusts in the tube and lead to obstruction. Finally, he will be unable to talk. To be deprived of the ability to communicate in the strange and often frightening atmosphere of an intensive care unit is a terrible thing, and the nurse will have to show great patience and sympathy in sustaining her patient during this difficult time. The keystone of tracheostomy management, therefore, is a meticulous tracheal aspiration technique, efficient humidification, and attention to the patient's psychological needs.

Aseptic technique must be observed during tracheal aspiration. Sterile gloves must be worn and a fresh, sterile catheter used for each aspiration. Gentleness is essential. If the tracheal mucous membrane is damaged, infection will enter and bronchopneumonia will follow. This complication is notoriously difficult to treat and is often fatal. It is significant that the organisms responsible are not those which are commonly found in the bronchial tree, but those which abound in the ward environment, in the bedding and in the hair, the nose and on the skin of the nurse. The inevitable conclusion is that infection has been introduced from outside during tracheal aspiration. Trauma to the mucosa must be reduced to a minimum. If a catheter, attached to a fierce vacuum source is pushed into the trachea, it will suck and tear at the mucous membrane. This effect can be reduced by inserting a plastic 'Y' connection in the vacuum line, so that suction is only applied when the nurse occludes the open limb of the 'Y' with her thumb. The catheter is passed gently into the tracheostomy tube as far as it will go. Suction is used only as the tube is withdrawn (Fig. 22). Suction catheters have been devised with special tips which do not suck and pull at the tracheal lining.

The anatomical arrangement of the main bronchi is such that the suction catheter passes into the right bronchial tree far more easily than into the left. If the head of the patient is turned well to the right, the catheter may be encouraged to enter the left main bronchus. This technique is equally applicable to aspiration through an endotracheal tube. The frequency with which aspiration must be performed should be judged from the needs of each patient; a rigid schedule should not be followed. Some patients with copious secretions will need aspiration every 5 or 10 minutes, others will need attention only every hour or two. Bubbling breath sounds are an absolute and urgent sign that secretions must be removed.

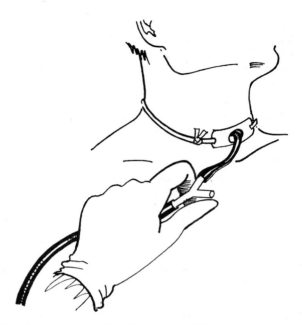

Fig. 22. Tracheostomy suction. Notice the 'Y' piece in the suction line so that suction is only applied when the thumb is placed over the open limb.

The above remarks about the management of the cuff of an endotracheal tube apply equally to the tracheostomy tube. It should be remembered that secretions and saliva tend to accumulate above the inflated cuff, as the mechanism which prevents swallowed liquid from entering the trachea is impaired in long-term tracheostomy patients. Hence tracheal suction should be carried out immediately after the cuff is deflated, and oral fluids should not be allowed unless the lungs are protected by an inflated cuff.

Modern plastic tracheostomy tubes have largely superseded the older metal types with their removable inner tubes and those made of red rubber. Tubes may need to be replaced from time to time, and this is made considerably easier if a flap tracheostomy has been performed. If a simple incision in the trachea has been employed, it will be necessary to use a tracheal dilator to hold the incision open when inserting the tube during the early post-operative days. Later a track will develop. If there is difficulty in passing a suction catheter and the neck becomes distended with air (surgical emphysema), assume that the tube has become dislocated into the space in front of the trachea. Under no circumstances should the tapes be tied with a bow at the back of the neck. The bow may be untied mistakenly during removal of an operation or X-ray gown, with fatal dislodgement of the tube. Tapes should be firmly tied with a reef knot at one side of the neck.

Specimens of tracheal aspirate should be sent for culture from time to time and antibiotic therapy given as determined by the sensitivity tests. As an additional safeguard against cross-infection, the outlet ports of mechanical ventilators may be connected to an exhaust system so that exhaled gases are not allowed to escape into the air of the unit.

Humidification

Humidification of inspired gases may be achieved by a variety of methods, few of which match the superb efficiency of the upper air passages, which can warm and saturate with water vapour the air inhaled on the coldest and dryest of frosty mornings. Perhaps the most effective, and certainly the most expensive, is the ultrasonic humidifier. Water is dripped onto a porcelain dish which is vibrated at ultrasonic frequencies, thereby shattering the drops into a dense fog of droplets. Care must be taken that this extremely efficient technique for delivering water to the respiratory tree does not result in over-hydration of the patient. Alternatively, the gases may be passed over a warm water bath interrupted by copper baffle plates. The Bird ventilator incorporates a nebulizer which works in the same way as a scent spray. Whatever form of humidifier is used, the moist gases are conducted to a plastic box which is fitted over the tracheostomy or to a 'T' shaped fitting which plugs into the tracheostomy tube. If none of these appliances is available, reasonable humidification may be obtained by instilling 2–3 ml of N. saline solution directly into the trachea every hour, or using a continuous slow drip through a very fine needle.

General management and aftercare

Finally, we must consider the question of communication between patient and nurse. A pencil and note pad should be provided, together with a handbell so that the nurse's attention can be attracted. The technique of weaning a patient from a ventilator is discussed in Chapter 5.

It is sometimes possible, if the patient is strong, to remove the tube and cover the tracheostomy stoma with a gauze pad. The patient is taught to press on the dressing with his finger if he wants to speak or cough. In older, weaker patients, particularly if the tube has been in place for a long time, the transition from life with a tracheostomy to life without must be made more gradually. The vocal cords have been idle for so long that the protective role of the glottis and the ability to speak may well have been lost. Such intermediate stages as the use of progressively smaller tubes with speaking valves or tubes with a hole cut in the elbow so that the stoma is maintained for aspiration of secretions but the patient is able to breathe in a normal fashion may have to be employed. Even when the tube has finally been removed, it will still be possible to pass a suction catheter through the tracheostome for some days.

MAINTENANCE OF PULMONARY EXPANSION

In health, the lung completely fills the pleural cavity, being separated from the lining layer of pleura by a thin film of lubricating fluid. The lung is an elastic organ, which tries to contract towards its attachment at the lung root. It is held in an expanded state against the chest wall in much the same way that a rubber sucker sticks to a window pane. There is a negative pressure in the potential space between lung and chest wall. If this space is entered by a knife thrust, or at operation, air is sucked into the chest and the elastic lung contracts into a small airless lump. Lung function may be impaired by either a collection of air (pneumothorax) or fluid within the pleural space (Fig. 23).

A collection of blood (haemothorax) may result from injury or surgery. Infection may be responsible for a clear effusion or pus (empyema); clear effusions may also complicate heart failure, malignancy and renal disease. Rarely, injury to the thoracic duct may lead to an effusion of milky chyle. The combinations of a pneumothorax with collections of clear fluid, blood or pus are respectively designated as hydropneumothorax, haemopneumothorax and pyopneumothorax. Whichever type of collection is encountered, compression of the lung will lead to breathlessness. The diagnosis is made by physical examination supplemented by

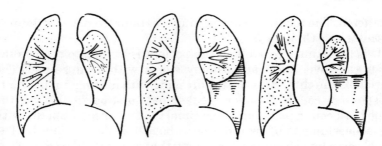

Fig. 23. (A) Pneumothorax; (B) pleural effusion; (C) pneumothorax with effusion.

radiography. The object of treatment is to secure full re-expansion of the lung by removal of the collection. This may sometimes be a matter of some urgency.

A pneumothorax may result from rupture of an air blister (bulla) on the surface of the lung. Air will enter the pleural cavity with each breath and be unable to escape because the ruptured bulla acts like a valve. As more and more air accumulates, the lung will collapse. In extreme cases the mediastinum will be pushed over to one side thereby embarrassing the action of the heart and compressing the remaining lung (tension pneumothorax). The acute breathlessness may be relieved dramatically by thrusting a wide bore needle into the chest. Air under pressure will escape and the crisis will be averted. Definitive treatment may now be started at leisure. The two techniques usually employed for removing fluid or air from the pleural cavity are aspiration with a needle and syringe and the insertion of an underwater sealed drain.

Aspiration of a pleural effusion

Although aspiration of a pleural effusion is a medical responsibility, the nurse should be able to lay up the trolley and prepare the patient. Needles should be of the trochar and cannula pattern (Universal or Martins needles). If a sharp pointed needle is used the lung may be pricked and a pneumothorax will result. A 20-ml syringe, three-way tap with a length of tubing which fits on to one arm and a large jug should be provided; a 10-ml syringe, a long needle, 1% lignocaine, towels and skin preparation solution complete the equipment. If the unit employs sterile packs, a very serviceable aspiration set can be assembled from disposable equipment. A short plastic intravenous cannula with stylet is an excellent substitute for the standard aspirating needle and plastic syringes and three-way taps are convenient and effective. If a large volume of fluid is to be removed, a wearisome task can be made considerably easier by using a Potain's aspirator.

There is no doubt that the most comfortable position for a patient undergoing a chest aspiration is sitting astride a chair with his folded arms resting on a pillow laid across the chair back. Most patients in an intensive care unit will not be well enough to get out of bed; if they are very ill aspiration should be performed with the patient lying in the lateral position with the side of the effusion uppermost. Alternatively he can be sat up and given a bed table with a pillow to lean on. This position is not well tolerated for long periods and is likely to produce cramp in the legs.

Intercostal tubes and underwater seal drains

The intercostal tube is one of the basic tools of intensive care, and yet its management worries many nurses who are nevertheless quite happy to handle complicated electronic instruments. This is surprising, as the principles are simple. If a general surgeon has to drain a collection of fluid or an abscess, he inserts a tube into the cavity and allows the contents to escape into a bag or into the dressings. If a similar tube is inserted into the chest, fluid will certainly escape, but air will be able to enter. The patient will develop a pneumothorax. This can only be prevented by some form of valve, which allows air or fluid to run out, but stops air entering the pleural space. Recently a valve has been devised which resembles a large party squeaker (the Heimlich valve), but the standard and almost universally used technique is to dip the end of the drainage tube below the surface of some water in a large jar. It is not difficult to see that this will prevent air from running up the tube into the chest while at the same time it permits fluid and air to drain. Furthermore, this device enables the volume of fluid drained to be accurately measured. We use 500-ml graduated measuring cylinders fitted with a rubber bung through which two holes have been drilled. A long length of glass or plastic tube passes through one of these holes to the bottom of the cylinder, which is filled with water to a depth where the end of the tube is about 1.5 cm below the surface. The volume of water is noted so that this can be subtracted from subsequent measurements of fluid drained. The second hole in the rubber bung is either left open or connected to a suction motor (Fig. 24).

The underwater seal drain is also, in effect, a water manometer which measures changes in pressure within the chest. As previously mentioned, the intrapleural pressure is negative, and this sucks a column of fluid up the glass tube to a height of about 5 cm. As the pressure in the chest varies with respiration, the column of water will rise and fall with each breath. The value of this observation is that it tells the nurse that there is no obstruction in the drainage tube. If the water in the tube does not swing, then the patient is either sitting on the drainage tube, or it is kinked in some way, or it has become blocked by blood or fibrin or the lung has become stuck over its end inside the chest.

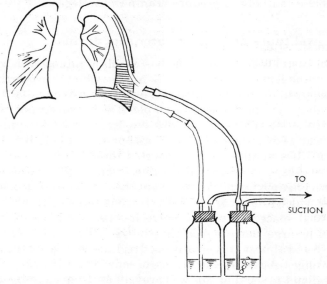

Fig. 24. Diagram showing intercostal drains being used to evacuate fluid and air from the pleural space. The underwater seal bottles have been connected to a suction pump.

Having assembled the underwater seal system a few simple rules must be followed in order to ensure that it functions efficiently:

1. The rubber tubing connecting the drainage tube to the bottle must be so arranged that the patient does not lie on it, that no dangling loops trail from the bed to the bottle and that the tubing does not kink where it is connected to the glass tube. This is done by supporting the tubing with a safety pin which picks up the sheet on either side of the tube. Of course, a pin must never be driven through a tube or air will leak in and spoil the water seal effect.

2. At no time must the apparatus be disconnected unless the tubing is securely clamped close to the patient's chest. If it does become disconnected accidentally, immediately fit it together again and encourage the patient to cough so that any air which may have entered the chest is expelled. It is wise to connect a sucker motor to the bottle to make sure that no pneumothorax remains. Then ask for a radiograph to be taken and summon medical help. Never clamp a bubbling chest tube for longer than is absolutely necessary or air will collect in the chest and the lung will collapse. The practice of clamping bubbling tubes while patients are transported from the unit to the ward or to the X-ray department is highly dangerous.

3. At no time must the drainage bottle be lifted higher than the patient unless the tube is clamped. Failure to observe this rule may result in the unsterile fluid in the bottle syphoning into the pleural cavity. This is particularly likely when patients are being transferred from bed to a trolley.

4. Never, under any circumstances, connect a patient to an underwater seal bottle unless you are certain that it contains water and that you have personally ensured that the drainage tube is connected to the long tube which goes under the surface of the water. It is surprising how often this elementary precaution is disregarded and anxious moments are spent trying to discover why a patient has suddenly become acutely breathless. The practice of having two lengths of tubing passing through the rubber bung, one long and one short, is usually to blame for the confusion. We have discontinued the use of the unnecessary short tube for this reason.

5. If considerable quantities of fresh blood are being drained the tubing will rapidly become blocked by clot unless it is milked frequently between finger and thumb. This can be very hard on the fingers unless the tubing is powdered with a little talc or a special milking instrument is used.

Insertion of intercostal catheters in the unit

When drainage tubes are inserted their number and exact position must be recorded in the notes so that there can be no confusion in the minds of the nursing staff. After open heart surgery it is usual to have one tube in the back of the pericardium and the other draining the anterior mediastinum. Mitral valvotomy and similar procedures which are performed through a lateral thoracotomy may have a single tube draining the base of the chest. After lobectomy or segmental resections of the lung it is usual to have two drainage tubes, one passing to the apex of the chest and one to the base. That to the apex is usually anterior to the basal, and there is more of it in the chest (and hence, less of it sticking out). It is as well to find out the habits of your surgeons in this regard so that there will be no confusion when the time comes to remove one or other of the drains.

Not infrequently intercostal catheters need to be inserted in the unit because the patient has developed a pneumothorax or because he has been admitted with a chest injury or there is a collection of blood in the thorax. The surgeon will need a trolley laid up with the usual towels and skin preparation solutions, a scalpel, skin suture, a pair of scissors and two pairs of forceps for clamping the tube. There should be a generous supply of 1% lignocaine and a 20-ml syringe and needle for its insertion.

The instruments used for passing a drainage tube between the ribs into the pleural space are a large trocar and cannula. The nurse should ensure that there is a sterile whistle tip catheter which is a snug fit in the cannula and can be pulled right through it with a firm tug (Fig. 25).

The usual site for insertion is either in the second intercostal space anteriorly or on the lateral aspect of the chest in the midaxillary line. After infiltrating the tissue planes down to the pleura with local anaesthetic, the surgeon makes a small incision in the skin and through this he thrusts the trocar and cannula, between the ribs and into the chest. The trocar is removed and the catheter is threaded through the cannula. The cannula is now removed, leaving the catheter in place. This is secured with a stitch or adhesive strapping.

A convenient alternative is now available, which consists of a plastic catheter with a disposable metal stillette (Argylle Co.). A trochar and cannula are unnecessary. The catheter is inserted through a short skin incision, and the stillette is then withdrawn.

Some surgeons favour the Heimlich valve, which takes the place

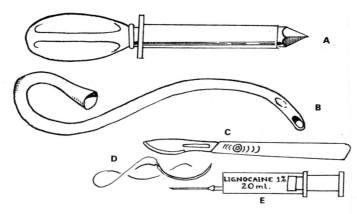

Fig. 25. Equipment for the insertion of an intercostal drain. (A) Trocar and cannula; (B) whistle tip catheter; (C) scalpel; (D) skin suture; (E) local anaesthetic.

of the underwater seal bottle. The valve is a rubber reed, rather like a party squeaker, contained in a plastic cylinder which fits onto the end of the intercostal catheter.

Use of suction apparatus

The vacuum lines to each bed station in the unit are admirable for the aspiration of secretions from the bronchial tree, but are too powerful to be connected directly to an underwater seal system. If they are to be used, a reservoir with a valve capable of controlling the negative pressure should be interposed between the vacuum point and the drainage bottle. Commonly, an electrically driven vacuum pump is used, and the pattern chosen depends upon the reason for which suction is being employed. If gentle suction is required to remove fluid or small quantities of air, the Roberts' motor will serve admirably. The suction is produced by two little pistons and cylinders; rather like a toy steam engine. It will be seen that such a system is capable of removing only a limited volume of air or fluid. If larger volumes are to be removed, as, for example, after lobectomy when large quantities of air escape from the raw surface of remaining lung tissue, then either a Matburn or Tubbs-Barrett pump is more suitable. These machines work on the principle of the cylinder vacuum cleaner, the sucking force being produced by a fan. Unfortunately, if they are used for prolonged periods continuously, the electric motors are liable to burn out.

The object of suction applied to an underwater seal system is to remove air from the pleural cavity as fast as it escapes from the surface of the lung. The lung will then remain fully expanded and, hopefully, will become adherent to the chest wall, thereby sealing the air leak.

You will be able to decide whether the suction motor is achieving this objective by looking at the pressure gauge. If it records a negative pressure, ideally about −3 mmHg, then the pump is winning the battle. If it is not able to produce a negative pressure, then air is escaping into the chest faster than the pump can remove it. Surgeons differ in their views about the use of suction. Some believe that it perpetuates air leaks by sucking air through ruptured alveoli and preventing them from sealing. Others believe that achieving full expansion of the lung will be the quickest way to stop air leaks. You should ask what the current practice in your unit is.

How to remove intercostal tubes

Tubes are removed simply by snipping the retaining stitch and pulling, but there is a risk that air may suck into the chest through the tube wound before the nurse can apply an occlusive dressing. It is desirable to have a positive pressure in the chest as the tube is pulled out in order to prevent this. Tell the patient to take a deep breath in and to hold it. Then pull. Some surgeons leave an untied skin suture through the wound. If you hold this with your left hand as you pull out the tube with your right, the edges of the wound will be held together, no air can enter and the suture can be tied at leisure. Alternatively, a pad of gauze backed by adhesive strapping can be quickly applied to the wound. The additional sealing properties of a petroleum jelly gauze are not really necessary, and such dressings tend to produce soggy wounds.

There is no mystery about the correct time to remove drainage tubes. There is no point in retaining tubes when they are no longer doing the job for which they were inserted. If no more air or fluid is escaping, they should be removed. It is profitless to leave a blocked tube in place. Tubes are painful things which tend to impede coughing. They should not remain in the chest for a day longer than necessary. You will be able to tell if a drain is blocked because the respiratory swing on the fluid level in the underwater seal bottle will stop.

MAINTENANCE OF VENTILATION— THE CHEST WALL

The ribs and the diaphragm act like bellows, sucking air into the lungs and blowing it out. We are not usually conscious of the work needed in order to do this, but if the lungs become stiff as a result of heart disease or certain lung conditions, breathing can become very hard work indeed. Breathlessness has been defined as consciousness of the need to do extra work in order to breathe. Observe a breathless patient. He uses almost every muscle attached to his chest wall to assist in the labour of forcing air in and out of the lungs. Muscles in the neck and abdominal wall contract, and in extreme cases the patient sits up gripping the edge of the bed so that he can use the pectoral muscles as well.

Estimation of blood gases

Respiration may be ineffective, either because chest wall movement is inadequate or because the lung is so diseased that the exchange of gases between the alveolar air and the blood is hindered. When this happens, the carbon dioxide content of the blood will rise and the oxygen content will fall. Two systems of measuring the oxygen and carbon dioxide content of the blood are in common use. The modern SI (*Systeme International*) units express these in kilopascals (kPa), the older system uses millimetres of mercury (mmHg). You will notice that both of these are units of pressure, which may seem an odd way of describing amounts of gas dissolved in blood. The concept is a little difficult to grasp. If you have a gas contained in a bag, it will exert a pressure on the walls of the bag. If the bag contains a mixture of gasses the pressure will be the same but each gas will be responsible for part of that pressure. The proportion of the pressure will be the same as the proportion of the gas by volume. For example, if the gas mixture contains 25% carbon dioxide, and the pressure on the wall of the bag is 100mmHg the 'partial pressure' exerted by the carbon dioxide will be 25mmHg. The same rule holds if the gas is dissolved in a liquid. The normal partial pressure of carbon dioxide in blood is 4.7–6 kPa (40 mmHg). If the mechanism for eliminating carbon dioxide fails, this will rise—in chronic bronchitic patients to as much as 11 kPa (80 mmHg) or higher. A PCO_2 above (45 mmHg) is taken as a definition of respiratory failure.

In the same way, the oxygen content of the blood will fall, and this may be measured in one of two ways. Arterial blood is normally 100% saturated with oxygen and the oxygen dissolved in the plasma exerts a partial pressure (PO_2) of 11.3–14 kPa (100 mmHg). If he were breathing pure dry oxygen the PO_2 would approach atmospheric pressure of 90 kPa (700 mmHg). In fact levels of 80 kPa (600 mmHg) are recorded. You will see that it is essential to know the concentration of oxygen in the inspired air if the results of PO_2 estimations are to be interpreted correctly.

Even though the PO_2 falls to 8 kPa (60 mmHg) the oxygen saturation of the arterial blood will still remain at satisfactory levels; greater than 80%. Once the PO_2 level falls below 8 kPa (60 mmHg) the blood rapidly becomes desaturated, and the patient will be in danger of death from hypoxia. As a very rough guide, a patient breathing room air should have a PO_2 of 13 kPa (100 mmHg), breathing 50% oxygen it should be 40 kPa (300 mmHg) and breathing 100% oxygen it should be 80 kPa (600 mmHg). Estimations of PO_2 should be performed on arterial blood obtained from an artery with a needle and heparinized all-glass syringe.

Any patient who is being treated with a mechanical ventilator or who may be in respiratory difficulties should have frequent estimations of blood gases as these determine the type of treatment needed and check that such treatment is being effective. Two other values are usually given when blood gas estimations are requested. These are the pH of the blood and the sodium bicarbonate content (standard bicarbonate). This is because the balance between carbon dioxide and bicarbonate ion is the principle mechanism whereby the acidity of the blood (pH) is maintained at a constant level. If the PCO_2 rises, the blood will become more acid (pH will fall from its normal level of 7.4). The acidity of the blood is expressed also as the hydrogen in concentration which is normally 36–43 mmol/l. In contrast to the pH, the value rises as the blood gets more acid. Any deviation in pH is very poorly tolerated. Blood may become more acid either because carbon dioxide is retained (respiratory acidosis) or because acid products of metabolism accumulate (metabolic acidosis). This latter condition is the sequel of a poor peripheral circulation such as is found in heart failure or hypoxia or renal failure. If the tissues are being perfused with a poor oxygen supply carried by a sluggish bloodstream the break-down of energy-producing material is incomplete and acid waste products are produced. Whatever the mechanism giving rise to acidosis, it can only be corrected by either eliminating the acids or by neutralizing them. The former is achieved by improving venti-lation, thereby blowing off the excess carbon dioxide or improving the circulation, thereby improving tissue metabolism. The latter is achieved by elevating the bicarbonate level of the blood and hence neutralizing the acids. The body may be able to do this naturally by reducing the amount of bicarbonate excreted by the kidneys, or it may be necessary for the surgeon to give bicarbonate as an intravenous solution. An 8.4 solution of sodium bicarbonate con-tains 1 milli-equivalent of the bicarbonate ion per millilitre. As much as 150–200 mEq may be given in the management of metabolic acidosis produced by cardiac arrest (see Fig. 30). In the SI units, bicarbonate is expressed in mmol/l. Fortunately the figures are the same for the older system which uses mEq.

Recognition of inadequate ventilation

The conditions described above which lead to sputum retention and impairment of coughing will also tend to prevent the patient moving his chest wall effectively. In addition to pain and weakness the patient may be under the influence of drugs, either self-administered in a suicide attempt or given by doctors. Relaxant drugs used during anaesthesia may still have some residual effect and potent analgesics tend to depress respiration. Muscular weak-ness due to myasthenia gravis, unconsciousness, head injury and mechanical disruption of the skeleton of the chest by trauma or surgery are further examples of the wide variety of conditions which may be encountered.

However, by far the commonest reason for respiratory failure in this country is chronic bronchitis and emphysema. Every winter our hospitals fill with these patients and respiratory units exist whose whole purpose is to deal with these and similar problems. The patient whose lung has been largely destroyed by bronchitis exists on a knife-edge. The additional burden of a chest infection or a small pneumothorax will be enough to send him into respiratory failure. Respiration must be supported mechanically until the precipitating factor has been treated. Blood gas estimations provide the most accurate and trustworthy assessment of respiratory function but much can be learned from observation. Note whether the chest wall moves in and out adequately with each breath. Carbon dioxide retention produces a hot, flushed skin, a bounding pulse and an elevated blood pressure in a drowsy patient. This is a late stage of carbon dioxide poisoning and no patient should be allowed to reach it in an efficient unit. Coma and a peaceful death are very close.

When ventilation becomes inadequate the keystone of treatment is to take over the work of breathing with a mechanical ventilator. This is discussed fully in Chapter 6.

IMPAIRMENT OF THE CIRCULATION TO THE LUNGS

Sudden obstruction of the circulation to the lungs by a pulmonary embolism may lead to collapse and death. Occasionally the patient may survive long enough to have the embolus removed surgically. The principle concern of the nurse is to guard against this catastrophe by preventing thrombosis of the deep veins of the calf. Deep vein thrombosis is common during and after surgery, especially in the elderly, the obese and the dehydrated, and particularly if patients are allowed to lie immobile in bed for long periods. Take care that the legs are not compressed by a firm edge—such as a long patient overlapping the end of a short bed. Encourage foot and ankle movements and frequent changes of posture. There is a good case for the use of routine anticoagulation therapy in those particularly at risk. The introduction of subcutaneous heparin as a routine preventative measure is claimed to be very effective in reducing the incidence of pulmonary embolism. Cough, pain in the chest on breathing and a little blood in the sputum signal the occurrence of a small embolus which may herald a massive one. Warn the medical staff; they will almost certainly want to start anticoagulation treatment.

A massive pulmonary embolus produces cyanosis and acute distressing breathlessness which, oddly enough, is a little relieved if the patient lies down. Commence oxygen therapy immediately and be prepared to start external cardiac massage if the carotid pulse disappears. While awaiting medical help ensure that cardiac stimulant drugs and the necessary equipment for setting up an intravenous infusion are available.

The use of the enzymes, streptokinase and urokinase to dissolve pulmonary emboli has been tried although there is some doubt of their ability to dissolve old, organized clot. It is given intravenously, ideally by a catheter in the pulmonary artery, and achieves its effects within a few hours. The principal complication is haemorrhage, and hence it is not advisable to use this drug within 5 days of surgery.

Some special problems

Post-operative care of patients undergoing pulmonary surgery

Everything which has been said in this chapter applies with particular force to the management of patients after resection of a lobe or segment of the lung. Remaining lung tissue must be fully expanded with a clear airway. A few special problems are associated with the removal of a whole lung (pneumonectomy). The object of post-operative care is to maintain the heart and mediastinum in the midline. As there is a negative pressure on the side of the remaining lung, this must be balanced by a similar negative pressure in the empty pneumonectomy space. This is produced by aspirating air until a pressure manometer connected to the needle shows a mean pressure of −5 cm of water. If this negative pressure is lost because fluid accumulates in the pneumonectomy space or because the air leaks through the bronchial suture line, the mediastinum will be pushed over to the side of the remaining lung (Fig. 26). The patient will become dyspnoeic. Relief is afforded by

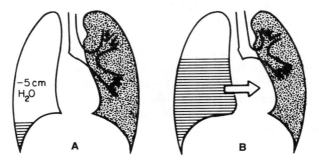

Fig. 26. Pneumonectomy. (A) Correct—with central mediastinum and negative pressure in pneumonectomy space; (B) incorrect—excess fluid in the pneumonectomy space has pushed the mediastinum over, thereby compressing the remaining lung.

aspirating air or fluid until the pressures balance once again. Many surgeons leave a tube in the pneumonectomy space, connected to an underwater seal bottle. It is usual to clamp the drain, releasing it for a brief period every hour. The aim of this precaution is to prevent an excessive quantity of air from being blown out of the pneumonectomy space when the patient coughs. This would result in the mediastinum being dragged across to the side of the operation.

Care of chest injuries

Chest injuries kill because of bleeding, drowning or suffocation.

Bleeding is particularly lethal if it is associated with hypoxia, as is usually the case in chest trauma. Blood is lost into the pleural cavity, which can easily accommodate most of the circulating blood volume, and also into the muscle layers surrounding the thorax. Immediate and adequate blood transfusion must be started as soon as the patient reaches hospital.

Drowning may be due to the accumulation of blood, sputum or vomit in the air passages. Rib fractures are painful and will impair coughing and deep breathing. Even a simple cracked rib may precipitate respiratory failure and sputum retention in an elderly bronchitic. The old method of strapping the chest restricts ventilation without easing the pain very much. Treatment is directed towards encouraging coughing and the relief of pain by analgesics or, sometimes, by blocking the painful area with a local anaesthetic.

Some centres use an indwelling fine catheter in the extradural space, through which local anaesthetic drugs may be injected.

Suffocation may be due to compression of the lung by air or blood collections in the pleural cavity, or because the skeleton of the thorax has been so damaged that it can no longer ventilate the lungs, or from lung contusion. Air and blood are drained by the insertion of an intercostal drainage tube. Minor air leaks from tears of the lung will usually seal; the rare major air leaks from rupture of a bronchus will require operative repair. Bleeding from the lung usually stops. All that is necessary is that the volume of blood drained should be measured and made good by transfusion. Severe, persistent bleeding is usually from vessels in the chest wall or the aorta or its main branches. This must be treated by early operation. Severe crushing injuries may produce multiple rib fractures. A large segment of chest wall becomes detached from the thoracic cage, and moves independently from the chest with respiration. It moves inwards during inspiration and is blown outwards during expiration. This 'paradoxical respiration' can be detected by a hand on the chest. It is immediately relieved by the administration of a relaxant drug, endotracheal intubation and manual inflation of the lungs. Currently, long-term treatment is by means of mechanical ventilation for at least ten days, until union of the fractures is sufficiently advanced to stabilize the loose segment of chest wall. A tracheostomy must be performed. Recently there has been a revival of interest in operative fixation of the segment (Fig. 27).

Contusion, or bruising of the lung, is sometimes called the crushed lung syndrome. The lung substance becomes an airless liver-like mass because of extravasation of blood into the tissue planes. This is managed by mechanical ventilation with a volume cycled ventilator, and many patients will recover after about three weeks of this treatment. In this, as in all thoracic trauma, frequent estimations of blood gases provide invaluable guidance. Antibiotics are used to prevent infection of the damaged lung. Massive doses of steroids are claimed to reverse the bruising process. Diuretics are also very effective in improving lung function.

Chest injuries are frequently associated with fractures of the spine, pelvis and limb bones and with head injuries. Rupture of abdominal organs and tears of the diaphragm may complicate the picture. However complex the injuries, the fundamental principles of maintenance of the blood volume and the prevention of hypoxia are of overriding importance.

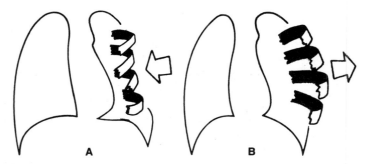

Fig. 27. Flail chest showing paradoxical respiration. (A) Segment drawn inwards during inspiration; (B) segment blown outwards during expiration.

Surgical emphysema

Air may escape into the tissues and under the skin if there is a pneumothorax and a breach in the chest wall due to either trauma or surgery. A swelling which gives a peculiar crackling sensation on palpation is characteristic. In extreme cases the whole body is blown up to a grotesque size, and the puffy eyelids prevent the patient from seeing. The condition is seldom dangerous. It is treated by removing air from the pleural space with an intercostal tube, and so preventing it tracking into the tissues. The most important part of the nurse's duty is to reassure the patient and his relatives.

Chapter 5
Mechanical Ventilation of the Lungs

Mechanical ventilation of the lungs is used today in a wide variety of circumstances. It is, however, important to appreciate that the need for artificial ventilation is not confined to patients who have actually stopped breathing, that is to say, who are apnoeic, but that it may be necessary also for patients whose breathing is still present but nevertheless is becoming increasingly inadequate for the maintenance of proper and effective gaseous interchange. In other words, it may be indicated in patients suffering from incipient but progressive respiratory failure. The increasing use of mechanical ventilation to support a failing respiration is one of the major advances in respiratory therapy in recent times, and an appreciation of the circumstances in which this rather drastic type of treatment is needed forms the background to learning the actual techniques involved in the management of patients who are undergoing a period of mechanical ventilation.

There are a number of conditions and circumstances where complete cessation of breathing may occur even when the heart is still beating and hence where the circulation is still effective. Respiratory depression to the point of arrest can occur, for instance, in response to the intake of respiratory depressant drugs either taken in overdose or administered as part of a general anaesthetic. Alternatively, apnoea can be a manifestation of a severe cerebral vascular accident and in both these situations prompt and continuing artificial respiration is necessary for as long as the precipitating cause is present. However, in contrast to these situations where breathing has stopped, a less acute form of respiratory failure can occur and where this is progressive it can result in a state of affairs in which although breathing is still present, the physical effort of moving air in and out of the lungs is becoming more and more exhausting for the patient, whilst at the same time the gaseous exchanges are becoming less and less

91

efficient. This state occurs with many severe and fatal illnesses involving disease of the lungs and it is in this group that the employment of artificial ventilation during the acute phase of the illness can be life-saving.

We need to consider in more detail these two groups of conditions in which it may be necessary to employ mechanical ventilation.

Respiratory arrest

The commonest reason for respiratory arrest in the presence of normal cardiac action is deliberate paralysis of the respiratory muscles by means of a muscle-relaxing drug of the curare type. This is commonplace in modern anaesthetic techniques and the facility with which anaesthetists today employ such drugs to abolish spontaneous breathing is an indication of the safety and effectiveness of artificial ventilation techniques when they are expertly applied.

In addition to the muscle-relaxants, however, respiratory depression to the point of apnoea can be produced by a wide variety of drugs including the opiates, barbiturates, tranquillizers and anti-depressants, but in spite of the fact that many of these drugs produce some measure of cardiovascular depression, they are all primarily 'killers' in overdose as a result of their depressant action upon breathing which in almost every instance will fail before the circulation does. Maintenance of artificial ventilation is, therefore, the principal and certainly the most important means of treatment for any patient who is suffering from the effects of an overdose of any drug which is primarily a respiratory depressant.

In addition to these chemical causes, breathing can cease from injury to the respiratory areas of the brain and brain-stem. Such injury may be the result of trauma or it may be a manifestation of pressure from a blood clot or effusion emanating from a cerebral haemorrhage or from the rupture of an intracranial aneurysm. In these instances, failure of breathing may precede cardiac failure by a significant and indeed often considerable period of time, and although prognosis in such cases is never good, there is no doubt that in some instances the brain damage is recoverable and that a period of artificial ventilation may be life-saving during the acute phase of the incident.

Respiratory failure

It is obvious that artificial ventilation is needed immediately in respiratory arrest. In progressive respiratory failure, however, where arrest has not yet occurred, the need can be equally great.

Progressive respiratory failure can be the result of inadequacy of many factors of which destruction of the lung tissue by disease is perhaps the most important. It can, however, also result from inadequate respiratory movements, inadequate pulmonary circulation or inadequate nervous or biochemical control of respiration.

Thus, respiratory inadequacy can be due to: weakness of the respiratory muscles; disease processes in the lungs; pain from fractured ribs; inadequate pulmonary circulation; or from failure of breathing due to disturbances of the central control mechanisms. The treatment of any of these may necessitate the use of artificial ventilation of the lungs.

Common examples of disease processes which can result in these failure mechanisms are as follows.

Respiratory inadequacy

Fatigue in severe debilitating illness
Peripheral neuritis and poliomyelitis
Residual curarization following anaesthesia
Multiple fractures of ribs
Abdominal pain in postoperative period

Disease processes in the lungs

Acute pneumonic illnesses
Acute bronchitis and asthma
Chronic long-standing and progressive lung disease
'Shock lung' (lung contusion)
Aspiration pneumonia

Inadequate pulmonary circulation

Cardiac failure
Pulmonary hypertension
Collapse of areas of the lung

Pulmonary embolism
Patients after cardiopulmonary bypass

Failure of breathing-control mechanisms

Poisoning of respiratory centre in the brain by drugs
Anoxia of the respiratory centre due to increased intracranial
    pressure
Disturbance of body chemistry
Respiratory centre failure following a period of cardiac arrest

This list is incomplete but serves as an indication of the wide
range of conditions which can necessitate mechanical ventilation
of the lungs. Furthermore, several of these conditions can be combined as when a patient with bronchopneumonia suffers from some
lung destruction, some collapse of lung areas, some heart failure
and a great deal of physical fatigue. Whatever the cause, however,
there may be a need—and often an urgent need—for artificial
ventilation for a period of time in order to support the respiration
whilst the patient receives more conventional treatments for the
causal conditions. The artificial ventilation will need to be continued until such time as these treatments have achieved their
desired results and then, and only then, can the patient be 'weaned'
from the ventilator and normal breathing re-established. Mechanical ventilation is, therefore, employed as an intensive therapy
procedure to support the vital function of respiration during the
acute and potentially fatal phase of the illness.

Mechanics of ventilation

It is important to realize that mechanical ventilation as carried out
by modern breathing-machines is largely a process whereby air or
air/oxygen mixture is forced into the lungs by a positive pressure
generated by the ventilator itself. Indeed, looked at broadly, a
ventilator is nothing more than a generator of positive pressure
which is then transferred to the patient's lungs in an intermittent
manner resembling normal breathing. The term applied to this is
intermittent positive pressure respiration—usually abbreviated
to IPPR.
    IPPR, although resembling normal breathing in that the lungs
are expanding and contracting rhythmically, is not exactly the

same mechanical procedure as normal breathing, which is essentially a suction effect whereby air is drawn into the lungs by the expansion of the rib-cage. This basic difference between normal breathing and IPPR is important since the substitution of the positive pressure inflation of the lungs for the suction effect of the expanding rib-cage influences the return of venous blood to the heart and, therefore, the cardiac output and the systolic blood pressure of the patient.

During normal breathing the expansion of the rib-cage on inspiration draws air into the lungs, but in addition the suction effect also helps to draw blood from the inferior vena cava into the right atrium of the heart. Since the cardiac output in any subject is proportional to, amongst other things, the venous return and the cardiac filling, reduction of these results in diminution of cardiac output and this may show as a fall in the systolic blood pressure. Any patient in whom IPPR is substituted for spontaneous breathing may, therefore, show a fall in systolic blood pressure.

The extent to which this disturbance of circulation develops will depend upon a number of factors, not least important of which is the degree of positive pressure being employed to inflate the lungs. Clearly the inflation pressure needs to be kept as low as possible compatible with producing the required degree of lung expansion. This expansion will be from the hilum of the lung outwards as the positive pressure is being applied via the trachea. Furthermore, the extent to which the lungs are being 'blown up' can be varied according to need, and the greater the inflation pressure used, the larger the amount of lung distension.

It should not be assumed that the greatest possible inflation will always benefit the patient, for this high distension which needs correspondingly high pressures will influence the venous return to a greater extent than more moderate ones, and hence cardiac output will be more likely to fall to dangerous levels. Inflation pressures in fact do not need to be higher than 15–25 cmH$_2$O in normal lungs, but where lung disease is present the lung tissue may be resistant to inflation and in such instances, higher inflation pressures will be necessary with consequent decrease in venous return. The ventilator produces a recurring pattern of intermittent positive pressure which is applied via the trachea to the lungs. In between inflations the pressure must fall back to atmospheric to allow the lungs to deflate by their own inherent elasticity together with the normal recoil of the chest wall.

The next point to consider, therefore, is how this rhythmic pattern of IPPR generated by the ventilator can be controlled so that the lungs are neither over-inflated nor under-inflated. The point at which a ventilator ceases to inflate and 'cuts out' in order to allow the lungs to deflate is known as the 'cycling point'.

Cycling

During the process of inflating a lung, the positive pressure employed raises the internal airway pressure above that of the atmosphere. In the normal adult lung full inflation will have taken place when this pressure reaches somewhere between 15 and $25\,cmH_2O$ (the exact pressure varies considerably from person to person). By allowing a ventilator to inflate to this pressure and then to cut out and allow the chest to deflate is one method of cycling. Machines which operate on this principle are known as *pressure cycled ventilators*.

An equally effective way of cycling a machine is to consider not the pressure inside the lung but the volume of air or gas which is being pushed in at each inflation. The normal adult tidal volume is between 0.5 litres and 1.0 litre per breath and hence it is possible to develop a machine which cycles by ceasing to inflate the lungs when a predetermined volume of air or gas has been introduced, and which then 'cuts out' to allow the chest to deflate as before. Such machines are known as *volume cycled ventilators*.

There is also a third principle upon which ventilator operation can be based. Inspiration and expiration take specific finite times. Inspiration at rest takes about $1\frac{1}{2}$ seconds, and expiration about $2\frac{1}{2}$ seconds. Expiration is followed by a pause after which inspiration again takes place. This timing of breathing allows a third method of cycling. Such machines are known as *time cycled ventilators*.

There are thus three mechanical ways in which any ventilator can be controlled and all machines incorporate at least one of these mechanisms. Some of the more sophisticated machines incorporate two and sometimes all three mechanisms, so that the most suitable one can be selected for any particular patient.

Triggering

In addition to the cycling mechanisms mentioned above there are occasions when it is desirable to allow some measure of spontaneous breathing by the patient but to assist this with a ventilator. This situation can arise under a variety of circumstances, for example, in a patient who is still partly under the effects of a muscle-relaxant drug but who is otherwise normal. Again in patients who have almost reached the point where IPPR is no longer necessary but who nevertheless still need a little assistance. Under these circumstances, some ventilators can be made to operate in response to the patient's own inspiratory efforts. The patient breathes at his own rate and each inspiration initiates or 'triggers' an inflation by the ventilator. Cycling at the end of this triggered inflation may be by any of the three aforementioned methods, i.e. volume, pressure or time, but the ventilator itself does not inflate the patient again until the next breath by the patient 'triggers' it to do so.

This patient triggering mechanism can be of value in the types of case mentioned and, in addition, it can be used in respiratory failure. The difficulty with this technique is that if the patient stops breathing altogether the ventilator will not 'blow' at all—for this reason the use of triggering has nowadays largely been replaced by the technique of intermittent mandatory ventilation (IMV), and this is described later in the chapter.

Which ventilator?

In some ways it is unfortunate that there are so many different makes and models of ventilators, since the choice of machine for any particular patient is more often than not based upon an individual doctor's preference rather than a specific patient need. There are, however, certain aspects of ventilator choice which are therapeutically important.

If the patient has normal lungs but requires artificial ventilation, any of the mechanical ventilators listed will be suitable. The choice is one of individual preference and availability. In such patients it is of little physiological importance whether the ventilator is pressure cycled, volume cycled or time cycled, so long as it is correctly set for the particular patient and is in efficient working condition.

When pulmonary or cardiovascular disease is present, however, it is of considerable importance to choose the most suitable ventilator. When high lung inflation pressures are needed—as in asthma and bronchitis—it is of advantage to use a ventilator which is either volume or time cycled, since pressure cycling mechanisms are less efficient and certainly less safe. Likewise, where cardiovascular failure is present and pressures within the chest need to be kept low, a pressure cycled ventilator set at low pressure may be desirable to impede venous return to the heart as little as possible.

The interpretation of patient needs in terms of 'which ventilator' can be simplified if we bear in mind the basic question—'Are the lungs normal?' If the answer is 'Yes', then the choice of make and type of cycling mechanism is relatively unimportant, and will depend upon the type of machine available and upon personal preference. If, however, the lungs are abnormal, then choice of cycling mechanism is important although choice of make and type of machine is again one of availability, provided the chosen model possesses the desired cycling mechanism.

In spite of these criteria, one commonly finds that workers in different intensive therapy units get used to certain machines and certainly nursing staff prefer to use the machine with which they are most familiar. This is a desirable state of affairs and too many machines of different types and makes will be avoided by wise unit directors.

Lung inflation patterns

The mechanics of lung inflation are highly complex but it is not essential here to study this problem in minute detail. It is necessary, however, to realize that the amount of resistance which a lung and a rib-cage can offer to inflation is extremely variable. The resistance to inflation offered by a normal lung with the subject fully under the influence of a muscle-relaxant can be as low as $15\,cmH_2O$, whereas it may not be possible to inflate a severe asthmatic with pressures of up to $60–70\,cmH_2O$. Lungs which inflate easily are said to have a good compliance, whereas lungs which offer difficulty are said to have poor compliance. Perhaps a better term would be resistance—thus lungs with good compliance offer a low resistance to inflation. Lungs with bad compliance offer a high resistance. In practical terms this means that the inflation pressure required by the lungs will also vary between one patient and another, and hence the control of the inflation pressure is one important aspect of ventilator adjustment.

There is a second factor regarding inflation which is important.

This is the pattern of inflation which the ventilator employs, and generally speaking, the most important aspect here is the speed with which the gas flows into the lungs. If there is little resistance to inflation, a predetermined volume of gas (the tidal volume) can be pushed into the lungs quite quickly. Hence in a normal relaxed subject it is quite easy, even with a relatively low inflation pressure, to push 900 ml of gas into the lungs in about $1\frac{1}{2}$ seconds. If there is resistance in the wall of the chest or in the lungs, as for example, in bronchial spasm, it may take more than double this interval to push in 900 ml of gas, even with a high inflation pressure. This is a physical phenomenon and can be compared to the effort required to blow through a narrow tube, which is always greater than that required to blow through a wide one.

In general terms, therefore, it will be necessary to use higher inflation pressures in diseased lungs than in healthy ones. Furthermore, a 'slow, steady blow' will always be more effective than a quick sharp one for inflating diseased lungs. These factors are taken into consideration when adjusting the ventilator settings, so that not only the inflation pressure but also the actual speed of inflation can be adjusted in the light of the patient's requirement.

Lung deflation patterns

Although all ventilators blow gas into lungs they do not generally suck it out. The recoil mechanisms of the lungs and the chest wall are normally utilized during expiration but here again there are mechanical factors which will influence deflation of the lungs.

Just as poor compliance can result in poor inflation—so too it can lead to poor deflation. Bronchial spasm may indeed offer greater resistance to expiration than it does inspiration, and where delayed lung deflation is a factor in patient ventilation, the length of time allowed for adequate expiration to occur must be increased. Thus the 'expiratory pause'—during which deflation occurs—must be lengthened, and again this is a necessary adjustment in the ventilator controls.

Negative phase

Under some circumstances it may be helpful if the ventilator can be made to 'suck' at the end of the expiratory period to produce what is known as a 'negative phase'. The introduction of a negative or subatmospheric phase can aid both lung deflation where this is slow, and venous return to the heart where this is impaired, either by circulatory collapse or by high inflation pressures. Negative phase is not used in routine mechanical ventilation, but is reserved for patients where its advantages are likely to be greater than its disadvantages. A negative phase can lead to collapse of areas of lung alveoli (with consequent non-inflation). It should be employed only after careful consideration of all the findings.

Blood which flows through a collapsed area will leave the lungs just as de-oxygenated as when it arrived. This blood will mix with blood which has been oxygenated in the non-collapsed areas and will thus reduce the total oxygen in the blood leaving the lungs. The process whereby blood fails to be oxygenated in the lung is known as 'pulmonary shunting'—a term which is often used in intensive therapy unit jargon.

Expiratory resistance

The opposite to negative phase is the situation in which a deliberate resistance to expiration is introduced so that the intrapulmonary pressure is never allowed to fall back to atmospheric. This results in a back pressure within the lungs—a situation which never occurs in normal breathing. The term applied to this technique is 'positive end-expiratory pressure' (PEEP). There are several reasons for introducing such an expiratory resistance and back pressure. Firstly, it may be done to elevate the central venous pressure and so reduce the risk of air embolus during operations upon the head and neck carried out in the head-up posture, and secondly, it may be employed as an empirical method of reducing pulmonary oedema in patients who develop cardiac failure during ventilation. In this instance, the 'back pressure' tends to prevent oedema developing in the alveoli. The commonest reason for introducing PEEP, however, is to hold the alveoli in an expanded state at the end of the respirator's expiratory phase, so avoiding collapse and shutting down of the alveoli and consequently improving oxygenation. The amount of PEEP can be varied according to the patient's needs but the usual range is between 5 and $10\,\mathrm{cmH_2O}$ and end-expiratory pressure. In severely diseased lungs the value of using PEEP is very considerable and the monitoring of the values of the end pressure is an important part of ventilator management.

Ventilatory management

The practical aspects of ventilatory management are based upon the factors described above, together with an understanding of the actions of specific drugs employed to facilitate ventilation, and to make this an experience tolerable for the patient. These patients are severely ill people and at all times they must be treated as such.

Patients undergoing mechanical ventilation fall into two groups; those who are unconscious and those who are aware of their surroundings. The first group—represented by patients with severe head injuries or drug overdose—are easier to manage as the conscious aspects of the situation do not arise—at least in the early stages. The second group—represented by patients after cardiac surgical operations and patients with severe lung disease producing respiratory failure—need, in addition to all the respiratory aspects, skilled management of their emotional state which will in most instances involve the use of sedative, tranquillizing and analgesic drugs.

A further factor in management will be whether or not any spontaneous breathing is present, thereby necessitating either patient cooperation with the ventilator or deliberate abolition of spontaneous breathing by relaxant and respiratory depressant drugs, so that the more efficient respiratory exchanges brought about by the ventilator can proceed without impairment by the patient's own inefficient efforts.

Basic principles of ventilator management

All patients who are undergoing IPPR will either have a cuffed endotracheal tube or a tracheostomy with a cuffed tracheostomy tube. All tubes should be of the plastic material type. Rubber and latex tubes should not be used for prolonged ventilation patients. The point at which this tube is connected to the hoses which come from the ventilator is always the weak link in the pressure circuit, and its integrity is a basic observation in ventilator management. If this connection becomes accidentally parted, the machine will cease to inflate the patient, and unless this is rapidly reconnected the patient will die of asphyxia. For this reason, patients undergoing IPPR must be under constant observation and the incorporation of a suitable ventilator alarm warning device is now regarded as standard procedure.

The adequacy of the ventilation of the patient needs to be assessed regularly in two ways; firstly, by clinical and secondly by biochemical measurement.

Clinical measurement

The amount of air or gas which is introduced into the lungs at each inflation of the ventilator is the *tidal volume* and the total of all the inflations each minute is the *minute volume*. The rate per minute and volume per inflation can be adjusted to give predetermined tidal and minute volumes. An average adult requires a tidal volume of about 900–1200 ml and a minute volume of between 9 and 12/lmin; however, patients can vary widely in their needs. These volumes can be measured by various types of ventilation meter, some of which are built into the ventilators. A commonly used separate instrument is the Wright respirometer.

Biochemical measurement

When the ventilatory volume and inspired gas composition is correct, the concentration of oxygen and carbon dioxide in the blood will be maintained within normal limits. The important measurements are the PO_2 and the PCO_2 and these are made by subjecting an arterial blood sample to blood gas analysis. Regular estimates of blood-gas values will, therefore, act as an accurate biochemical control of the adequacy and efficiency of ventilation. The normal value for the PCO_2 is 5.1 kPa and a good working rule is to try to maintain the level at just below this. There will, however, be circumstances when figures both below and above this are acceptable in the light of the clinical condition of the patient. The value of the PO_2 will also be estimated at the same time and the normal figure for this value is of the order of 12 kPa.

Humidification

All patients who are undergoing IPPR need humidification of the inspired gases unless the period of ventilation is brief, as during the course of an anaesthetic. Failure to humidify the inspired gases adequately leads to drying and crusting of the mucus in the trachea and bronchi so that it can not be aspirated. Techniques of humidification vary from infusion of saline via a drip into the trachea, to sophisticated ultrasonic nebulizers. All ventilators used for prolonged ventilation incorporate humidifiers and these should always be used. Care should be exercised, however, to ensure that too much fluid does not accumulate in the ventilator hose and that in the case of heated humidifiers, that the temperature is kept within the recommended limits.

Bronchial toilet

Periodic bronchial toilet is an essential part of ventilator management. The frequency with which it needs to be carried out in any individual patient will depend upon circumstances. Hourly toilet and bag inflation of the lungs should be regarded as the standard practice. The technique of what is colloquially called 'bagging and sucking' warrants detailed description as it is a very vital part of management, and it is in this area that physiotherapist and nurse cooperate most fully together in intensive therapy unit work. The intensive therapy unit aspects of physiotherapy are specialized and require special skills. The nursing staff need to be equally skilled in these techniques and physiotherapist and nurse should be complementary and interchangeable in this situation.

'Bagging and sucking'

The regular inflation of the lungs by the ventilator will be at a predetermined rate and volume, which once instituted change but little unless either a deliberate alteration is made, or the patient's pulmonary state alters significantly. It is, however, desirable that from time to time a very full expansion of the lungs should occur. This in fact does occur in normal breathing. It is known as the 'sigh mechanism' and is specially noticeable during sleep.

Deliberate hourly expansion of the lungs by means of a manual breathing-bag accompanied by bronchial lavage and suction, should take place in all patients undergoing IPPR, and whilst the frequency can vary greatly, most patients will benefit if a 4 hourly routine is adopted. The patient should be disconnected from the ventilator and the lungs should be well inflated by hand. This should continue for one or two minutes during which time intermittent bronchial suction is applied. The extent of this 'bagging and sucking' will vary according to need. In some patients it may need to be done frequently. On the other hand, in patients who are

tired, ill and exhausted, it may be kinder to allow several hours'
sleep even at the expense of some reduction in ventilatory efficiency.

Bronchial toilet accounts for a great deal of the activity of the
staff in a busy intensive care unit if several patients require IPPR.
It must never be neglected. Furthermore, a high standard of sterile
technique is essential—hence the need in all intensive care units
for a high nurse-to-patient ratio. Sterile gloves, gowns and masks
must be worn if any infection is present and although the cross-
infection hazard can be reduced by isolation, the main protection is
always good nursing discipline and cleanliness. Isolation of
patients, although theoretically the ideal, requires a higher staff-
to-patient ratio and is probably less effective in preventing cross-
infection than is generally believed, *unless* it is accompanied by a
high standard of nursing discipline.

Certain hazards can arise during these bronchial toilet procedures and especial care should be taken to ensure that the
suction catheters are always sterile, and that they are supple
enough to pass down into the main bronchi without traumatizing
the delicate mucosa. At the same time they should be sufficiently
rigid to stay patent even with high suction pressures, and not
collapse down at the time when they are supposed to be collecting
secretions. Full sterility with no-touch techniques should be employed during bronchial toilet.

Excessive lung inflation with the manual bag technique can also
be potentially dangerous as venous returns and hence cardiac
output can be temporarily impaired if pressures are too high.
Inflation at these times should be full, but not greater than that
necessary to expand the lungs completely and hence enable secretions to drain down into the main bronchi where the suction catheter can reach them. It is during this procedure that the
physiotherapist employs her special techniques to assist drainage
of secretions.

Pneumothorax

The possibility of rupture of part of the lung and consequent
pneumothorax must be borne in mind, especially when high inflation pressures have to be employed. It is almost impossible with
modern ventilators to rupture a normal lung, but where disease is
present, certainly small leaks and sometimes large ones, can

develop. The development of a pneumothorax represents one of the hazards of IPPR in diseased lungs and a close watch needs to be kept for any such complication. Disappearance of 'breath sounds' as heard with a stethoscope over the chest together with a patient who in spite of apparent chest inflation appears hypoxic, are the characteristic signs of this serious complication. The immediate treatment consists of releasing the pressure within the chest by the introduction of a large bore needle followed by the introduction of an underwater drain to avoid recurrence.

Drugs and sedation

Patients who are comatose, commonly from head injury or drug overdose, will rarely require additional drugs to facilitate mechanical ventilation. Patients who are conscious, however, will almost always need some form of medication to enable them to tolerate, both physically and emotionally, the considerable stresses of IPPR.

Sedation

Foremost amongst the patient's needs will be sedation to allay apprehension and to facilitate rest and sleep in the presence of the ventilator and its accompanying endotracheal connections. Unless unconscious from another cause, all ventilator patients require some sedation. Diazepam is a drug which is especially valuable since it can be given intravenously in doses of 10 mg without inducing hypotension. Furthermore, it can be repeated as necessary at frequent intervals. Other drugs, which have a place include lorazepam and papaveretum BP which will also act as an analgesic and a respiratory depressant. The need for tranquillization and rest is a very important and, unfortunately, an all too frequently overlooked patient need, in a busy intensive care unit. Omission is a serious error of management and there is today rarely any excuse for such lack of patient understanding, as the range of drugs available is wide and their safety margins are great.

Analgesics and depressants

Primarily, one is concerned here with analgesia for pain together with depression of the cough reflex, but actual depression of spontaneous respiration in order to facilitate IPPR is also of importance. All the opiates are of value but perhaps the most valuable drug is phenoperidine, which has high analgesic and respiratory depressant properties, and can be safely combined with diazepam. Dosage will be of the order of 1.0–4.0 mg intravenously as necessary, to depress breathing, and caution should be shown with the early doses as hypotension can occur. Generally speaking, this drug is effective and safe in most patients, but some individuals appear resistant to its depressant properties. In these cases it is better to employ muscle-relaxants than to use larger doses with a risk of hypotension. An alternative drug to phenoperidine is fentanyl which has a similar action but of shorter duration. The dose of fentanyl is 0.1–0.4 mg intravenously. Papaveretum BP in doses of 5.0–10.0 mg i.v. is also a valuable agent.

Muscle-relaxants

Where sedation and respiratory depressants do not allow unhampered IPPR or where muscle resistance is a problem, as in tetanus, one or other of the long-acting muscle-relaxant drugs can be used. D-Tubocurarine, alcuronium or pancuronium are all suitable drugs but since they do not have any inherent sedative and analgesic properties, it is necessary to combine them with one or more sedative and analgesic drugs to make the paralysed state less stressful. It is of interest to note, however, that where good ventilation is practised and where PCO_2 levels are kept below 3.8 kPa, there is usually little awareness present except during the times when bronchial toilet is being carried out. It must be borne in mind that unless sedation is heavy, patients under the influence of the relaxants are able to hear what is said and to appreciate pain without being able to react to either situation.

The management of patients who are undergoing a period of artificial ventilation is, therefore, a combination of technical expertise in ventilator adjustment, the employment of a range of sedative, analgesic and relaxant drugs and, above all, an understanding of the patient's emotional and nursing needs. No aspect of nursing can be forgotten; the specialized knowledge of respiratory problems is always additional to basic nursing care, and must never be allowed to replace it as the prime consideration. The good intensive therapy nurse must start by being simply—a good nurse.

The inspired gases

All patients undergoing IPPR should be inflated with a mixture which contains a proportion of air, and the use of pure oxygen is potentially dangerous except for brief periods of time, as for example when 'bagging and sucking'.

The admixture with air is essential for two reasons: firstly because the inclusion of nitrogen in the air helps to maintain alveolar expansion and secondly because prolonged ventilation with high inspired oxygen concentrations leads to fibrotic changes in the lungs. This is known as 'oxygen toxicity'.

The concentration of the inspired oxygen in the mixture can be calculated either from the flows of air and oxygen which can be measured, or by the interposition of an oxygen analyser into the breathing circuit just before the gases reach the patient.

The actual concentration of oxygen in the arterial blood can, however, be measured by blood gas analysis and such analysis is now a routine in all patients who are on IPPR. The normal PO_2, breathing air, is about 12 kPa and during IPPR this figure may vary widely according to the degree of lung damage and to the concentration of oxygen in the inspired mixture. The working rule should be to keep the figure as close to 12 kPa as possible.

With very damaged lungs arterial oxygen levels well below 12 kPa may be found even with high oxygen levels in the inspired mixture, and it is in such cases that the use of positive end-expiratory pressure (PEEP) is of very considerable value as it allows reduction in the inspired oxygen levels with consequent lessening of the dangers of oxygen toxicity.

Weaning

When the period of artificial ventilation has served its purpose, it becomes necessary to terminate the procedure and restore natural breathing. In many instances, this poses little problem but, in some patients—more especially those who have undergone IPPR for a prolonged period—a period of gradual weaning is necessary. Weaning can vary between merely discontinuing ventilation and allowing the patient to breath spontaneously, to more gradual weaning over several days during which periods of IPPR by the ventilator alternate with spontaneous respiration. In intractable cases where lung damage of a more permanent character is present, the weaning period can be lengthy and it is especially during this time that the ability of the nurse to encourage and reassure the patient is of immense value.

Aids to weaning

There are three methods whereby weaning from the ventilator can be assisted. These are:

1. Increased dead space technique
2. Continuous positive airway pressure (CPAP)
3. Intermittent mandatory ventilation (IMV)

Increased dead space

The stimulation of respiration by CO_2 is well known and if the patient's dead space is artificially increased by means of an extension piece to the endotracheal tube or the tracheostomy, the increase in CO_2 accumulation will act as a respiratory stimulant and allow the PCO_2 to rise (Fig. 28). It is important to monitor the PCO_2 levels during weaning, but it must be borne in mind that in patients with chronic respiratory disease the 'normal' PCO_2 may

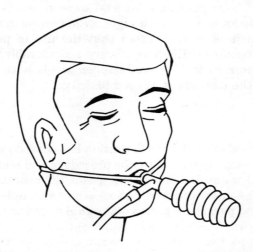

Fig. 28. Extension piece fitted to endotracheal tube to increase dead-space. This is used when weaning a patient from a mechanical ventilator.

be much higher than in the healthy patient, and for these patients spontaneous breathing is only possible if the CO_2 is higher than normal. Levels of the order of 7 kPa are not uncommon in chronic respiratory disease.

Continuous positive airway pressure

Continuous positive airway pressure or CPAP as it is usually referred to, is an extension of the principle of PEEP to the patient who is breathing spontaneously.

The principle here is that the endotracheal tube or the tracheostomy are connected by a 'T' piece to a widebore hose through which a high flow of humidified air-oxygen mixture is passing. The outlet end of the hose is passed to an underwater seal and the depth of the water determines the amount of positive pressure created in the widebore hose. The spontaneously breathing patient has therefore to breathe out against this water pressure.

CPAP can be a valuable aid to weaning especially where lung damage is present and alveolar collapse is likely, but it always necessitates either an endotracheal tube or a tracheostomy.

Intermittent mandatory ventilation

Intermittent mandatory ventilation is a more complicated technique and is of value when more simple methods of weaning have proved unsatisfactory.

The principle of IMV is one which combines some spontaneous respiration by the patient against CPAP with an occasional inflation of the lungs by a ventilator. The circuitry can be complex and requires careful setting up but the method is of great value in patients who have been on IPPR for long periods of time.

A tracheostomy, although not mandatory is usually present, and the successful use of the IMV technique requires a well motivated and cooperative patient. A variety of ventilators can be used and the main item of equipment in the circuit is a special IMV valve which can be fitted into a variety of different circuits.

Ventilator alarms

Most ventilators today are used with one or other of the proprietary ventilator devices which indicate either failure of the machine, disconnection from the patient or obstruction of the airway. There are many such alarm devices on the market and they are valuable aids to management of IPPR patients. Their principal value is to the nursing staff whose attention is drawn to a circuit which is defective by the loud buzzer on the alarm. Such alarms, however, have their limitations and although they will indicate that there is a defect in the circuit they will not specify what it may be.

In all cases, however, the availability of a rebreathing bag and a separate oxygen outlet by the bedside will ensure that manual ventilation can be adopted until the problems of the ventilator have been resolved. The 'bag by the bed' is the Intensive Care Unit's piece of life saving equipment *par excellence*.

Chapter 6
The Maintenance of Body Fluids and Electrolytes

There is still much confusion concerning the management of the hydration and nutrition of patients who are unable to eat or drink. Human bodies, like all other organisms, are complex packages of aqueous solutions which can be divided into several compartments. Under normal environmental conditions, with adequate access to food and water, a very fine balance is maintained between the contents of each compartment and between the whole body and the external environment. Disease states frequently change the internal and external balance and it is here that the therapist exercises his skills.

Units of measurement

Before discussing fluids and electrolytes, it is essential that the units of measurement are defined clearly and uniformly. Water is the largest single constituent of the body. It is convenient to measure its volume in millilitres. Rapid changes in body weight are usually a reflection of water gains or losses. A kilogram gain in a few hours represents the retention of a litre of water.

The water within the different compartments of the body contains chemicals called electrolytes. There is an equal number of chemical units (millimoles) of the positively charged cations (Na^+ K^+ Ca^{++} Mg^{++}) and the negatively charged anions (HCO_3^-, Cl^-, HPO_4^{--}, SO_4^{--}, organic acids, proteins) in body fluid. The strength of the solutions making up the body fluids is measured in milliosmols, which is the sum of the particles (ionized or nonionized) in the solution. Electrolytes are substances which split into positively and negatively charged particles (ions) when in solution, e.g. one sodium chloride molecule yields two ions, Na^+, Cl^-. Other substances exert an osmotic effect when in solution but are not ionized (e.g. glucose). By expressing weight in kilograms,

111

volume in litres, electrolytes in milliequivalents and solutions strength in milliosmols, calculations are simplified, balances are easier to evaluate and fluid and electrolyte shifts become clearer.

Normal fluid, electrolyte and food balance

The input of water, electrolytes and food is normally by mouth. The size of the intake is regulated by thirst, appetite and habit. When the excretory mechanisms are functioning normally these are completely satisfactory in maintaining health. Individual intakes vary with body size, physical activity, age and climatic conditions. In temperate climates the average 70-kg man undergoing moderate physical activity consumes 2500–3000 calories, 2000–2500 ml of water, 75 mmol Na^+ and 75 mmol K^+ each day. At least half of the water intake is not drunk but comes from the food (its contained water plus water of metabolism). It follows, therefore, that a patient who is not eating has halved his normal water intake even though he drinks normally.

Although a patient can survive without a calorie intake for several weeks, fluid deprivation causes symptoms in the healthy in a matter of hours and leads to death in a matter of days. The precise timing varies with the environment and the health of the patient and depends on the fact that the external surface of the patient is permeable to water. Even without obvious sweating, approximately 1000 ml are lost daily through the skin and lungs. These losses are greatly increased by fever and gross sweating. They are also greatly increased by rapid breathing and the breathing of dry air or gases. This is because each time a breath is taken the inspired air becomes saturated with water vapour at body temperature. The colder and drier the inspired air and the higher the patient's temperature, the greater the water loss. Dry gases are normally administered during anaesthesia and humidification of inspired air for patients on ventilators is often very inefficient.

Water and electrolytes are also lost in the urine. In health there is a powerful regulating mechanism to preserve water in situations of 'drought' and to excrete the excess when waterlogging is a danger. The normal urine volume, which depends on intake, is in the range of 600–1500 ml daily. When the urine volume is less than 600 ml daily the normal kidney is unable to excrete adequately the solid waste products. Diseased or damaged kidneys require a much larger urine volume to do the same job. Only small quantities of water are lost in normal faeces (Table 1) but diarrhoea is a frequent cause of excessive fluid and electrolyte loss.

The normal sodium intake varies widely from person to person, dictated largely by habit and taste. The addition of salt in food preparation and at table often leads to an intake three- or four-fold above that which is necessary for health. In the presence of heart disease, renal disease and hypertension, 'normal' sodium intakes can be dangerous.

Table 1. Normal ranges of water gains and losses.

Gains	Range (ml)	Losses	Range (ml)
Fluids	500–1700	Water vapour loss from skin and lungs	850–1200
Water in solid food	800–1000	Water loss in urine	600–1600
Water from oxidation of food and body tissues	200–300	Water loss through faeces	50–200
Total	1500–3000		1500–3000

The normal potassium intake comes from food and some drinks (e.g. beer). Except in the presence of severe renal failure potassium overload is rare. On the other hand potassium deficiency is seen in patients on long-term diuretic therapy who have not been given an extra potassium intake.

Abnormal fluid balance

The commonest imbalance in fluid management results from an inadequate intake. For example, if a patient is ill and does not eat but continues to drink normally, he, of necessity, halves his fluid intake. Therefore, in order to give an adequate fluid intake by mouth to a patient who is not eating, it is necessary to give 150 ml (a cupful) every hour for 17 hours a day. This gives the patient only 5 hours uninterrupted sleep. To achieve this, skilled nursing attention is required.

Although drinking is the most satisfactory way of maintaining an adequate fluid intake, it is often not possible for patients undergoing intensive care to drink. The patient may have disordered function of his gastrointestinal tract with vomiting paralytic ileus or diarrhoea, or he may be unable to swallow because of unconsciousness or paralysis. Under these circumstances the choice must be made between giving fluid via an indwelling gastrointestinal tube (nasogastric, gastrostomy, jejunostomy) or parenterally through a vein.

The next commonest cause for fluid and electrolyte deprivation in a patient in the ICU is abnormal loss of gastrointestinal fluids. This can be in two forms, external loss and internal redistribution or sequestration. The magnitude of the latter, which may take the form of oedema, cellular overhydration, ascites, pleural effusion or haematoma, is sometimes not recognized. The former is very much more dramatic, presenting as vomiting, diarrhoea or fistula loss.

Another equally dangerous common abnormality of fluid and electrolyte handling is seen when the excretory mechanism is unable to cope with the intake, for example, in patients with acute or chronic renal failure (see Chapter 7), cardiac abnormalities (see Chapter 2), and in the malnourished (see below). This condition may be aggravated by the injudicious administration of fluid and electrolytes by the therapist. The skilled therapist gives enough and no more and nursing assistants make frequent accurate observations to guide him. This is an important role of the ICU nurse (Fig. 29).

Observations required to manage fluid and electrolyte intake

It is a sorry situation that even today very few ICU patients are nursed so that changes in the major body compartments can be measured. Regular accurate measurements of body weight give a much more reliable estimate of fluid changes than any other method but weigh beds are rarely used for ICU patients. Regular weighing on chair or foot scales is very satisfactory for fit patients but is rarely possible when the patient is very ill. The alternative method of checking the hydration of an ill patient is to record the fluid gains and losses on a standard balance chart. As most patients in intensive care units will not be eating it is an easy matter to calculate the fluid intake (drinks, i.v. fluids, etc.). Accurate recording of fluid loss is more difficult. It is a relatively easy matter to measure urine output (with or without the use of a urethral catheter) but the collection of abnormal gastrointestinal losses (vomit, diarrhoea, fistula) is considerably more difficult. To these measured losses must be added the estimated volume of insensible loss through the skin and lungs. As we have discussed before, this is in the region of 1000 ml in most hospitals in temperate countries. This estimate can produce considerable discrepan-

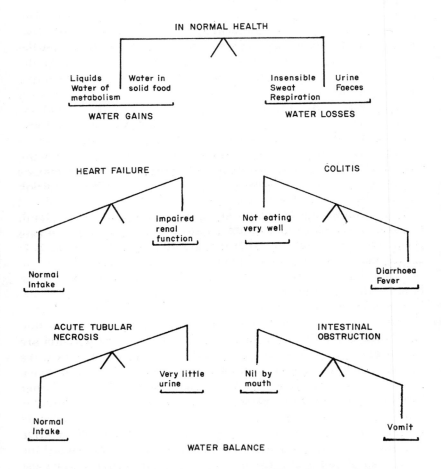

Fig. 29. In normal health there is a very delicate balance between intake and output such that total body water remains constant. Some disease states which affect this delicate balance leading to overhydration or dehydration are illustrated. Treatment is designed to restore the balance.

cies in the ill patient when taken with inaccuracies in other volume measurements, especially when there is renal failure. To be of maximum assistance to the medical staff it is essential that the nurse should record accurately all fluid losses and gains.

The composition is as important as the volume of fluid lost and gained. The intake of an ICU patient who is on oral or tube feeding should be supervised by a trained dietician so that the sodium, potassium and calorie intake is known. Such supervision also ensures that adequate vitamins are given. The composition of the intravenous fluids is easy to determine by reference to the labels on the bottles. It is often of great help to the therapist to record the amount of sodium, potassium and calories given to check with the prescribed intake.

Intake requirements are largely dictated by output. This can be calculated from a knowledge of the sodium and potassium content of the vomit, diarrhoea, fistula fluid and the sodium potassium and urea concentration in the urine. These measurements should be obtained daily from the clinical chemistry laboratory. The laboratory results are useless, however, if the samples are not collected and labelled accurately.

From a knowledge of the intake and output cumulative or serial balance graphs of water, sodium, potassium, etc., can be made and these are very helpful in therapy. Similar records of urea and creatinine excretion give valuable information on renal function. So far we have not mentioned serum biochemical changes. This is because they are rarely of much value without a knowledge of the intake and output of the patient. Blood urea, serum creatinine, sodium and potassium should be measured regularly. Serum creatinine estimations in conjunction with its urinary excretion give a good guide to renal function. Blood urea and urinary urea excretion additionally give an indication of the patient's catabolic rate. A rising blood urea may suggest dehydration. A low blood urea and low urea excretion may suggest hepatic dysfunction.

Low serum sodium may suggest overhydration and a high sodium either sodium overload or dehydration. A high potassium may suggest renal failure and a low potassium indicates a profound total body potassium deficit as may be seen in chronic diarrhoeal states or after prolonged use of diuretics.

Fluid and electrolyte replacement

1. *Methods of replacement*

The ideal way of receiving food and drink is by mouth. When this fails the most common method is the intravenous route. During the past 20 years the introduction of plastics and disposable equipment has made i.v. therapy much safer.

Intravenous drips. Even though the plastics have removed much of the chemical irritation effect on the veins, a recent report found that 48% of intravenous catheters were infected at the time the drips were removed. In this study, considerably more care was taken of the puncture site than is usual.

When a new intravenous infusion is being established, the nurse should ensure that the resident has the facilities and assistance to use 'full' non-touch technique. It is only by this means that the local and systematic infective complications of intravenous infusion therapy can be minimized. This is particularly important when catheters are being inserted into central veins or the vena cavae. This is often a tense situation for the resident and tactful help is invaluable. In patients who are being maintained intravenously for many days or weeks, septic venous thromboembolism from drip catheter is too frequent to allow for any complacency at the time of their insertion.

Percutaneous cannulation of veins has now largely replaced cut down drip insertion. This means that the vein can be used for a drip at a later occasion. Care should be taken that the plastic cannulae do not snap off and pass into the circulation. If they do they rarely cause symptoms. If a cannula does snap off and pass out of the limb and is symptomless it should be left alone. Much more harm is likely to come from searching for it in the heart or lungs. In the event of mechanical complications such as this, the medical staff should be notified as a matter of urgency. A drip that leaks into the tissues, or that is in a vein that has thrombosed, should be removed immediately as there is nothing to be gained by leaving it *in situ*. The nurse should use her tact to dissuade the new resident from inserting a drip into an anatomical site that will be inconvenient from the nursing standpoint. Ideally it should be possible to stabilize the cannula without resort to splinting the limb. In the very ill, who may need to be maintained intravenously for some time, it pays to be economical of drip sites. The site of needle insertion should be covered by a gauze dressing. Particular care should be taken to avoid contamination of the drip circuit when a three-way tap is used. Occlusive caps should always be used over the exposed portal. One-way injection ports are available on many cannulae and have done away with the need for three-way taps in most situations.

Peripheral veins are not satisfactory for the infusion of hypertonic fluids and intravenous food as they very rapidly thrombose. These preparations should always be given via large central veins. Leaving catheters in large central veins may lead to intracaval thrombosis and possibly infective thromboembolism. For these reasons it is still often preferable to hydrate and feed a patient through an indwelling tube in the gastrointestinal tract if at all possible. Three routes are commonly used—nasogastric, gastrostomy and jejunostomy.

Nasogastric tubes. Before the introduction of the modern plastic nasogastric tubes, gastrointestinal intubation was often complicated by severe side effects due to inflammation alongside the tube. This resulted in sinusitis and nasal, laryngeal and oesophageal ulceration leading to stricture formation. Unduly stiff tubes resulted in gastric perforation. Fortunately the plastic tubes do not cause these effects. They may, however, render the laryngeal and gastro-oesophageal sphincters incompetent. The presence of a tube may encourage gastro-oesophageal acid reflux and subsequent aspiration of gastric contents into the respiratory tract. The presence of a tube also stimulates the swallowing reflex. This encourages the entry of air into the stomach and beyond unless it is frequently aspirated. Under normal circumstances the volume of air swallowed is about the same as the volume of food and drink. The presence of a tube often doubles the volume. Gaseous distention leads to abdominal discomfort, and interferes with gastrointestinal function. Distention may also place undue strain on intestinal suture lines and abdominal incisions.

Gastrostomy. A gastrostomy can be performed under local anaesthesia or the tube may be inserted at the time of laparotomy. The anterior wall of the stomach is sutured to the anterior abdominal wall and a self-retaining balloon catheter is inserted. This may have a long limb beyond the balloon which can be passed through the pylorus into the small bowel. This method of intubation has many advantages over nasogastric intubation; in particular, it is more comfortable and does not make the gullet sphincters incompetent. Its insertion does require an operation and may lead to an infected area on the abdominal wall, especially in the malnourished patient with poor healing ability. It is useful for patients with pharyngeal and oesophageal lesions requiring protracted therapy.

Jejunostomy. This method of feeding is not very commonly used but still has a place in diseases proximal to the pylorus. It has all the advantages and disadvantages of gastrostomy. A balloon catheter is not used as this would cause intestinal obstruction.

2. *Types of fluid used*

There are very many different types of fluid available for intravenous administration. They are basically of two kinds—simple and compound. In modern practice there is little place for compound fluids as it is extremely difficult for the therapist to know precisely what he is giving his patient. More and more intravenous rotas are being prescribed from a small range of standard solutions. Let us examine the standard daily requirement for a patient with no abnormal losses in vomit, faeces (diarrhoea), fistula, etc.—2500 ml water, 75 mmol Na^+, 75 mmol K^+. This can be provided by 500 ml normal saline and 2×1000 ml dextrose to each of which 20 mmol K^+ as (KCl) has been added.

Normal saline (0.9% sodium chloride). It can be given intravenously or subcutaneously where it induces no inflammation and minimal swelling. It is prudent to use this as the first bottle in any drip therapy as it causes no reaction should there be a leak at the venepuncture site.

Dextrose (glucose). This is a convenient way of administering water intravenously. The 5% solution is isotonic. If pure water were given intravenously the plasma would be rendered hypotonic and red cell lysis would result. The dextrose is metabolized but as each bottle contains only 25 g it yields only 100 calories—this is too insignificant an amount to be dietically important. Dextrose is irritant to veins and leads to thrombosis. More concentrated dextrose, 50%, provides more calories, but is too thrombogenic to be given through a peripheral vein. It is valuable given into a central vein with sufficient insulin to control blood sugar levels. Fructose has become less widely used as it is often not metabolized.

Dextrose 4.3%, 1.5 N. saline. An alternative way of providing the same intake is to use five 500-ml bottles of a solution of 0.18% Na Cl and 4.3% dextrose.

Potassium. The older compound electrolyte solutions contained very variable amounts of potassium. Nowadays the pharmacy provides bags with the potassium content clearly marked. This reduces the chance of bacterial contamination when potassium was added in the ward or ICU. Only very rarely should more than 40 mol be added to a 1000 ml unit because of the risk of cardiac arrest (see Chapter 3), but in the ICU it may be necessary to give more concentrated potassium solutions. When this is being done the ECG should be observed carefully.

Bicarbonate and acid base balance

The pH of the plasma and extracellular fluids of man and most mammals is 7.4. One way the body has of regulating the internal pH or acidity is by the selective excretion of anions or cations in the urine. Another is by the excretion of carbon dioxide through the lungs. These two systems are superimposed on a system of buffers in the plasma. When there is an accumulation of acid products above what can be excreted it is necessary to support the buffering system of the plasma by bicarbonate or lactate. The former is most commonly given as sodium bicarbonate. A convenient way of administering this substance is as 1 mmol Na per ml solution. The amount required to neutralize a particular degree of acidosis can be calculated from the estimations of PCO_2, pH, standard HCO_3 with a normogram. Severe metabolic alkalosis, as is sometimes seen after prolonged loss of gastric juice, may be treated by administration of sodium chloride; the kidney excretes the excess sodium. On occasions ammonium chloride can be given but this is rarely necessary (Fig. 30).

ACID BASE BALANCE

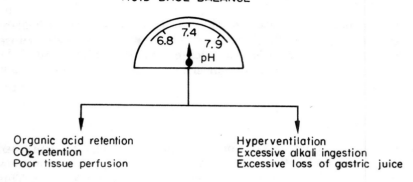

Organic acid retention
CO_2 retention
Poor tissue perfusion

Hyperventilation
Excessive alkali ingestion
Excessive loss of gastric juice

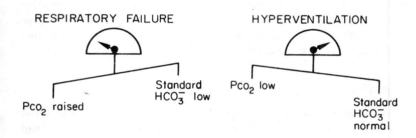

RESPIRATORY FAILURE

Pco_2 raised

Standard HCO_3^- low

HYPERVENTILATION

Pco_2 low

Standard HCO_3^- normal

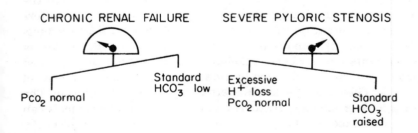

CHRONIC RENAL FAILURE

Pco_2 normal

Standard HCO_3^- low

SEVERE PYLORIC STENOSIS

Excessive H^+ loss
Pco_2 normal

Standard HCO_3 raised

Fig. 30. Acid base balance in the plasma: The pH of the blood is delicately balanced by the buffering system of the blood but can be changed by excessive rises or falls in carbon dioxide or organic acids.

It is useful to measure the pH, standard HCO_3 and PCO_2 to aid the treatment of seriously ill patients. Four illustrations are given of common abnormalities which are discussed further in the relevant chapters.

Other electrolytes

Except in long-term situations it is rarely necessary to consider the administration of other ions although theoretically a case can be made out for magnesium and calcium and zinc replacement. This is a subject which will not concern the nurse and is outside the scope of this book.

Intravenous diet

The same cannot be said for intravenous feeding. A nurse may appreciate better than the medical staff that an ICU patient is often starved. When ICU management is prolonged, starvation can be a potent factor in causing death. Until relatively recently, patients who were ill received very little calorie intake and this was mainly as carbohydrate. In some circumstances, as is discussed in Chapter 7, patients with renal failure were deliberately starved of protein. The main limitation of parenteral feeding was the inability to give adequate calories in a reasonable volume.

Carbohydrates

Concentrated sugar solutions can be used as a source of calories if given into a central vein. They sclerose peripheral veins. This action can be utilized in the injection treatment of varicose veins or haemorrhoids. 5% dextrose (see above) is a poor calorie source but 50% glucose is useful. Ethyl alcohol (ethanol) is sometimes used to provide carbohydrate calories. It is present in several proprietory mixtures for intravenous feeding and has the advantage of making the patients more cheerful. Some of the higher alcohols such as sorbital are undergoing evaluation as a source of carbohydrate calories. They must be administered into large veins to minimize the risk of thrombosis and their role in therapy has as yet not been fully evaluated. Carbohydrates provide 4 calories per gram.

Fats

The problem which delayed the progress of intravenous feeding for years was the difficulty in producing a fat emulsion which was stable in the bottle and in the bloodstream. Lack of stability of the emulsion in the bottle limited the availability of the fat. Lack of stability in the bloodstream led to fat embolism. A product which has proved extremely useful in clinical practice is an emulsion of soya bean oil in lecithin (Intralipid). This provides 8 calories per gram, and does not cause phlebitis.

The serum of patients receiving Intralipid must be observed for the presence of hyperlipaemia. It is usually not possible to administer more than 1000 ml 20% Intralipid daily without hyper-lipaemia. This has been held to be responsible for platelet damage, bleeding diatheses and acute renal failure. Current intravenous feeding régimes usually limit Intralipid to 500 ml 2–3 times weekly.

Amino acids and proteins

The third energy source in an oral diet is protein. The administration of protein intravenously is limited by the production of anti-bodies and consequently allergic and anaphylactic reactions. Therefore, for practical purposes, only human plasma proteins can be given intravenously to man. Supplies of these are extremely limited and expensive. They are indicated where there is a specific deficiency of a particular protein (e.g. albumin in liver disease, anti-haemophylic globulin in haemophilia).

For providing protein intravenously usually we must rely on supplying the amino acid building blocks from which protein is constructed. Several proprietary amino acid preparations are available. They are all mixtures of different substances. In general they contain all the essential amino acids and some of the non-essential ones. Recently new mixtures of amino acids have been introduced which include a high proportion of essential amino acids in the L-form and a low proportion of non-essential amino acids and D-forms. The mixtures may also contain other calorie sources such as glucose, fructose or ethyl alcohol. The sodium and potassium content of the preparations also varies and must be taken into account when ordering an intravenous diet. Most solutions give about 1 kcal/ml with 5–12.5g N_2/l.

Vitamins

There are generally enough vitamins in the body stores to enable a previously fit patient to survive a severe illness without developing vitamin deficiency. However, if the patient is malnourished before operation he is likely to be vitamin deficient. The body stores of the water-soluble vitamins B and C are the first to be depleted. The post-operative period without normal food only makes the deficiency worse. This deficiency can make itself apparent by poor wound healing (vitamin C lack) or an acute confusional state (vitamin B lack). Two or three injections of the BP preparation of intravenous vitamins is sufficient to correct any deficiency. Vitamin A and D deficiency (fat soluble) is very rare as the body stores are large.

Method of giving an intravenous diet

It is necessary to give intravenous food through a cannula in a large vein as peripheral veins rapidly become occluded. They should be inserted with full aseptic technique as casual technique will lead to a septic thrombophlebitis of the large veins or even the vena cava. This complication has not infrequently led to the death of these ill patients. Care should be taken if substances are added to intravenous feeding solution as precipitation may occur.

Using intravenous fat, amino acids, glucose and alcohol it is possible to give a 3500 calorie diet in a reasonable fluid volume (3000 ml). Although the latter three substances can be mixed in a bottle, fat cannot be added. If the individual bottles of fluid are given in series the serum levels of the constituents (sugars, amino acids, etc.) fluctuate widely and may easily excede the renal threshold. This results in the loss of valuable calories as glycosuria and aminoaciduria. Glycosuria may be controlled by the administration of insulin. This also controls the hyperosmolar state of the blood. It has been found that there is better utilization of the administered calories if the Intralipid, amino acids and sugars are run in parallel. This is performed by infusing them through drip tubing with a 'Y' connection (Fig. 31). It is probable that such a system causes less phlebitis than the same substance in series. There is evidence to suggest that the needs of the ward patient who requires intravenous feeding but who has normal renal, hepatic and pulmonary functions are different from the ICU patient who is often ill. The common ICU patient who needs intravenous feeding is acutely ill with perhaps shock, septicaemia, multiple trauma complicated by renal, hepatic or pulmonary failure.

For example a ward patient would be adequately managed by 2.5–3.0 l of compound amino acid, sorbitol, alcohol solution

(1000 kcal 5 g N_2/l) daily plus supplements of sodium, water soluble vitamins, calcium, potassium and phosphate as required.

An ICU patient would be better managed by an amino acid glucose régime giving the equivalent calories together with vitamins and trace elements. Insulin is required to maintain the blood sugar in the range 8–10 mmol. Hypoglycaemia must be avoided or cerebral damage will occur.

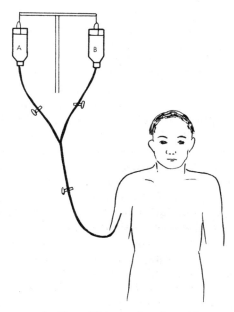

Fig. 31. Intravenous feeding. The two bottles of intravenous food are connected in a 'Y' position to a proximal vein preferably in the upper limb. This reduces the problem of thrombosis.

Sorbitol and alcohol are likely to induce lactic acidosis in the ill patient. Intralipid is better tolerated by the ward patient and is probably best avoided in the ill ICU patient. The fluid volume necessary to give adequate calories is a limitation in the use of intravenous feeding in renal failure patients.

In many hospitals the pharmacy make up the intravenous 'diet' for the patient in one bag for 24 hours and thereby reduce the risk of contamination of the fluids by additions made in the ICU or ward.

Tube feeding

Even though the cost of intravenous food has been reduced over the past decade it is still an expensive form of treatment. There remain very definite indications for its use. The patients should either be malnourished or likely to become so if not fed intravenously. Feeding should not be instituted during an acute crisis in an ill patient where more appropriate treatment might be fluid and electrolyte replacement or blood transfusion. Intravenous feeding should not be instituted if feeding by the gastrointestinal tract is possible. It is much cheaper, easier and safer to give a fluid feed down a nasogastric or enteric tube if this is at all possible. It is rarely necessary to resort to a feeding jejunostomy. When using tube feeds into the gastrointestinal tract absorption of water should be tested first by comparing the volumes given with those aspirated. If this is satisfactory, dilute milk, normal milk and high calorie liquid feed should be introduced in that order, and 12–24 hours apart. Diarrhoea may be a complication of this type of tube feeding but often responds to a less rich mixture. Another cause of diarrhoea is infection of the tube feed. The dietetic department or pharmacy usually provide nasogastric feeds in a sterile form. The days of the nurse with the liquidizer are over. Another serious complication of tube feeding is over-distension of the stomach with regurgitation into the pharynx and subsequent aspiration into the tracheobronchial tree. This complication is minimized by frequent aspiration of the tube to check for gastric retention. The problem is that the holes in the distal end of the tube tend to become blocked with food, which leads to a false sense of security.

Interpretation of biochemical and laboratory results

There should be a very close relationship between staff of the intensive care unit and the investigative laboratories to get the best service for the patients. The bridge between the two is very largely made by the nursing staff of the ICU. It is important that the nursing staff should be aware of the type of specimens that are required for a particular test and make certain that the sample is taken from the patient in the appropriate fashion. This may require a certain amount of tact in helping the new resident working in the unit.

There are very many types of specimens sent to the laboratory.

Some require urgent attention in the laboratory to give results which alter the patient's treatment (PO_2, PCO_2, pH, HCO_3^-, K^+, Hb, urea). Others are equally important when assessed serially over a period of time (Ca^{++}, urea, PCV etc.). You will note I have included urea under both headings. The degree of urgency must be conveyed to the laboratory at the time the sample is taken to help the technicians to produce the result soon enough. Here a telephone call each way is very helpful.

Often serial samples are taken in the ICU. It is important that they are correctly labelled so that the progress of the patient is known accurately, for example the order of blood-gas samples when weaning a patient from a ventilator or the difference between pre- and post-dialysis urea determinations. Although it is the medical staff who will alter treatment as the result of a laboratory test it is the duty of the ICU nurse to inform the doctor when the result is available. The nurse must appreciate the urgency of reporting such information. When should she telephone the doctor and when is it safe to leave discussion of the results to the morning or evening ward round? The nurse is in minute-to-minute contact with the patient and the doctor may well be dealing with patients elsewhere. To aid judgement it is useful for the nurse to know the normal values of the common investigations (electrolytes, haematology, etc.). This is aided by displaying the normal ranges in a prominent position on the unit notice board. A list of normal laboratory values is given on page viii.

Laboratory results are only valuable if they are available to the therapist. We find it very useful to record the results on a variable time base flow chart with some of the results shown graphically. The latter method is the clearest way of showing trends (blood urea, sodium excretion etc.). For example after renal transplantation we display the serial results of urea, haemoglobin, creatinine, urine proteins and urine volume of a patient to show recovery from tubular necrosis rejection episodes and the subsequent return of normal renal function.

Effect of trauma, surgery or other stress on fluid balance

Many large books have been written on the alterations in the control of water and salt excretion in stress. All that can be done here is to give the briefest outline of some of the more important events. An accident or operation acts as a stress to the patient.

Among other things it causes stimulation of the adrenal medulla with the outpouring of adrenaline, and of the adrenal cortex with increased secretion of the mineralocorticoids (aldosterone) and glucocorticoids (cortisol). The magnitude and duration of the response in the neuro-endocrine system depends on the magnitude and duration of the insult to the patient. The following are three examples of the many effects that can be observed soon after injury.

1. There is stimulation of the posterior pituitary gland via the hypothalamus which releases antidiuretic hormone. This markedly reduces the volume of urine excreted. This effect can be minimized by adequate fluid replacement and as such is a useful self-regulatory mechanism. It does, however, on occasions reduce the patient's ability to excrete excessive fluid volumes.

2. Increased secretion of aldosterone causes a reduction in the excretion of sodium ion by the kidney. This is again basically a protective action but may be responsible for salt (and water) overloading if large amounts of sodium ion are given soon after injury.

3. Increased secretion of glucocorticoids switches the patient into a catabolic state where he uses his body tissues as an energy source and is unable to use food to restore his flesh. This effect occurs maximally in the few days after injury or operation and is largely responsible for the weight loss which occurs at that time even in the face of a seemingly adequate diet. Even a patient who has had a straightforward repair of a hernia goes into this catabolic state for a few days. After a major procedure such as for ruptured aortic aneurysm or multiple fractures, the weight loss is much greater. Only after the first few days is it possible to reduce the breakdown of body tissues by feeding the patient. It is for this reason that intravenous feeding is not usually started for 5 days after operation or injury.

Chapter 7
Renal Function and its Importance in the Intensive Care Unit

It is only possible to describe in outline how the kidney works but it is important to be acquainted with this to understand the way that damaged kidneys influence the treatment of patients.

In health the kidneys:

1. Remove waste products from the blood (e.g. urea, uric acid, creatinine)

2. Regulate the internal chemistry of the body (e.g. sodium, acid-base balance)

3. Regulate the amount of water in the body

4. Help to regulate the blood pressure (renin)

5. Help to control red blood cell formation (erythropoietin)

6. Vitamin D metabolism

All these functions are vital to life and any impairment of renal function may influence the treatment of a patient in the intensive care unit.

Anatomy

The two kidneys are situated retroperitoneally high in the abdomen. Their upper part is protected by the lowest ribs. The receive their arterial blood supply from the upper abdominal aorta, usually from two main arteries, although multiple arteries are common (25%). The blood passes in a branching system of arteries within the kidney to supply arterioles to the glomeruli. There are about 1 million glomeruli in the normal human kidney. They are invaginated spheres leading to the renal tubules and lie in the superficial or cortical part of the kidney. After leaving the glomerular capillaries, the blood passes towards the deeper medullary part of the kidney to a second set of capillaries around the tubules. From there it passes to the renal veins.

The renal tubules, which transport the glomerular filtrate, can be divided into parts. The first part is the proximal convoluted tubule which is located in the cortex. The tubule then plunges into the medulla as the loop of Henlé and then upwards to the cortex again as the distal convoluted tubule. Finally it passes into the medullary pyramid as the collecting tubule. These fuse with each other before opening into the renal calyces which join to form the renal pelvis. This is connected to the bladder by the ureter.

Physiology

As the blood passes through the glomerular capillaries it is filtered. The filtrate enters the proximal convoluted tubule in the first stage of its passage towards the pelvis. During this passage there is selective reabsorption of substances such as water, sodium, potassium and the excretion of substances such as hydrogen ion into the urine. The activity of the renal tubule is under the influence of the antidiuretic and other hormones. It is very susceptible to ischaemic damage but has a remarkable capacity for complete repair following such damage. The renal glomeruli are less susceptible to ischaemic damage but when they are damaged they are not capable of repair.

Types of renal failure

Under most circumstances the normal kidney can cope with gross abnormalities of fluid and electrolyte intake or abnormal losses by preferentially excreting or retaining water and salts. It is only when the function of the kidney is impaired that special measures must be taken by the therapist. Three types of renal impairment are commonly seen in patients undergoing intensive care: *acute* renal failure, *acute on chronic* renal failure and *chronic* renal failure. It is important that a diagnosis should be arrived at early because the treatment of these conditions varies.

Diagnosis of renal failure

Let us first consider how to arrive at a diagnosis of renal failure. From what has been discussed in Chapter 6 it will be remembered that a normal urine output ranges from 600 to 1500 ml daily. A reduction of urine volume below 600 ml daily should be regarded as *oliguria*. When the daily urine volume fails to reach 200 ml the patient is *anuric*. Total anuria (zero output) is a relatively uncommon situation.

A diminished urine output is most commonly the result of an inadequate fluid intake for the particular circumstance of the patient even though the total fluid intake may be normal (2500 ml daily). For example, a patient with large intestinal losses (diarrhoea or vomiting or tube suction) may have an abnormal loss of 5–6 litres daily. Therefore, the first stage in the assessment of a patient is to review the fluid intake and losses (particularly the abnormal losses) of the preceding few days. These, together with a clinical evaluation of the state of hydration of the patient, give a very good guideline to management. For example, if the period of anuria is short (a few hours) and the patient is certainly not overhydrated, a fluid load of 1–2 litres should be given and the urine volume over the next 3–4 hours measured. Often the increase in urine flow is very gratifying. On occasions with a dehydrated patient 8–10 litres of fluid are needed to produce a sustained urine flow, but even then a response is usually seen after 1–2 litres have been given.

The second most common cause of pre-renal oliguria is inadequate perfusion of the kidney. The production of urine is an active process in the kidney and requires the presence of metabolically active cells. When the arterial perfusion of the kidneys falls below a variable minimum, urine production ceases. A fall in systolic blood pressure below 80 mmHg is a common cause for absent urine flow. There are two components to urine production, glomerular filtration and tubular function. If the hypotension is short-lived, raising the blood pressure allows filtration to restart before ischaemic damage to the tubules occurs. Longer periods of ischaemia cause necrosis or death of the renal tubular cells. Kidneys vary in their sensitivity to damage but there is evidence that minor degrees of damage go unnoted in clinical practice. A systolic blood pressure below 80 mmHg for more than 1 hour or complete obstruction to blood flow to a kidney at body temperature for 30 minutes may result in acute tubular necrosis. It is important to appreciate that some patients will develop acute tubular necrosis without a recognized period of hypotension. For example a young patient was transferred to our renal unit after a road accident in which he received multiple fractures. He received 3 units of blood although he had an injury which should have received 7 litres of blood. Despite this at no time was he hypotensive. His blood pressure had been maintained by adrenal medullary activity at the expense of adequate tissue perfusion. Radiologically it can be demonstrated that adrenaline causes intense renal artery spasm. Acute tubular necrosis is a recoverable lesion in the kidney but it may take several weeks for function to improve sufficiently to maintain life. Occasionally the blood supply to the kidney is impaired even further and this results in acute renal cortical necrosis which is often irrecoverable. This latter lesion is seen in association with pregnancy and when the renal arteries are blocked by emboli or thrombosis on atheromatous plaques. Venous obstruction to the kidney most commonly results in the nephrotic syndrome rather than oliguric renal failure.

Primary renal causes of acute renal failure usually take several days or a few weeks to cause oliguria. They are often secondary to some previous renal pathology (glomerulonephritis). They are usually suggested by the patient's history and are confirmed by subsequent investigations.

Anuria due to obstruction to urine flow is seen in patients in intensive care units. In conditions of unconsciousness retention of urine can be missed easily. Obstruction to urine flow may follow traumatic or surgical damage to the ureter, bladder or kidney. These cases can be identified by cystoscopy and retrograde urography.

Oliguria or anuria are not necessarily present in renal failure. Patients with severe chronic renal failure may produce a normal or even excessive urine volume. It may happen that the diagnosis of chronic renal failure is made on entry to hospital with an intercurrent illness. Care should be taken not to rely on an adequate urine volume to indicate adequate renal function.

What action should be taken when a patient becomes oliguric?

1. Check hydration state clinically
2. Check previous fluid intake and output
3. Correct hypotension which is a common cause in the ICU patient
4. If clinically normal or dehydrated, give a test water load
5. If over-hydrated give a diuretic (e.g. frusemide)
6. Make sure all intake and output are controlled
7. Check serum and urinary chemistry
8. If in doubt check anatomy of drainage system (cystoscopy, ascending urography and isotope renography)

9. Renal biopsy is sometimes indicated when the cause of anuria is not clear

10. Institute management of renal failure with fluid, salt and food intake control

What happens to a patient with acute renal failure?

Unless strict control of the fluid intake is instituted an anuric patient will become severely over-hydrated at the rate of 1–1.5 kg/24 hours. His excretion of urea and other metabolites will cease which will cause the blood urea to rise by approximately 6 mmol/l/24 hours. Unless an adequate supply of non-protein calories is provided, the urea rise will be much higher. In patients after surgical operations or trauma the rate of blood urea rise can increase to 3–4 times normal. This is due to catabolism of the body tissues. When this occurs the intracellular cation K^+ is released and the serum K^+ rises. If the serum potassium rises above 7.0 mmol/l there are dangers that the heart may arrest in diastole. Hyperkalaemia is often heralded by high T waves on the ECG. The acid base balance shifts to a metabolic acidosis but the buffering homeostatic mechanisms tend to minimize the change of pH.

A diet was devised some 30 years ago to counteract these changes. It consisted of a restricted water intake supplemented with sugar and fat to spare protein catabolism and potassium release. It was often called 'Bull's milk' after the originator. Although effective for short periods, it was very unpalatable and led to starvation. It has now been abandoned in favour of dialysis.

What is dialysis?

Dialysis is a way of altering the body constituents by placing a semi-permeable membrane between the blood and the dialysate fluid. Two types of membrane can be used: the peritoneum and an artificial membrane such as cellophane or cupraphane.

A model of haemodialysis can be created by suspending a cellophane bag containing blood in a glass of salt solution (Fig. 32). The blood is separated from the dialysate by the semi-permeable membrane. The pore size prevents egress of cells and large molecules like proteins into the dialysate but allows smaller molecules (e.g. glucose, urea, etc.) and ions (e.g. H^+ OH^- Cl^- Na^+ K^+ etc.) to pass through the membrane so that an equilibrium is reached across the membrane. In this way waste products like urea, water and potassium can be removed and substances such as glucose, HCO_3^- etc., can be gained by the blood. Changes in the concentration of the chemicals in dialysate have very important effects on the concentration of the substances in the blood but bacteria, fungi and viruses do not enter the blood. The modern haemodialysis machine also performs two other functions both of which cause a net loss of water from the patient. The total solute content of the dialysate is above that in the plasma so water is removed by osmosis. The pressure in the blood compartment is above that in the dialysate compartment so water is removed by ultrafiltration.

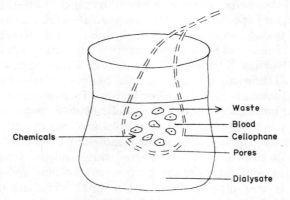

Fig. 32. The principle of dialysis. If a semi-permeable bag (cellophane) containing blood is suspended in a salt solution (dialysate), water, lower molecular weight molecules and ions pass through the membrane at a speed determined by the concentration of the substance. Larger molecules such as proteins and cells do not pass into the dialysate. All kidney machines use this principle.

Peritoneal dialysis uses the peritoneum as the semi-permeable membrane but in this case to avoid peritonitis the dialysate must be a sterile solution. Haemodialysis requires a sophisticated machine to circulate the blood across a membrane which is bathed on the reverse side by the dialysate.

Peritoneal v. haemodialysis

These are both efficient, clinically useful methods of treatment but each has its limitations. Peritoneal dialysis is unable to cope with the metabolic processes of a highly catabolic patient (e.g. after severe injury or major operation). It is also difficult to manage in a patient who has intra-abdominal pathology or adhesions after previous operations. Although peritonitis is not an absolute contra-indication to peritoneal dialysis and is a good way of administering antibiotics, gross abdominal distension may make this method of management difficult and distressing to the patient. Chronic peritoneal sepsis, pain and loculation of the fluid by adhesions often limit the time available for this treatment. It may, however, be used for many months.

Haemodialysis is more satisfactory for long-term use. The clearance rates of the dialysers are adequate to cope with even the highest catabolic rates. Access to the circulation in the short term can be accomplished by two venous cannulae (which need to be in big veins). This method is now rarely used except in emergencies. The most usual method of cannulating patients with acute renal failure is through a Teflon silastic arteriovenous shunt. For long-term treatment recurrent needling of the varicosities produced by a surgically created subcutaneous arteriovenous fistula is the usual method. The insertion of a shunt is a tricky surgical procedure. The presence of the tubing gives rise to chronic low grade sepsis around the insertion tracks which may lead to thrombosis of the shunt. Shunts can be declotted by sucking out the clot. However, shunts may work satisfactorily for many months or even years.

Nowadays most patients with medical types of acute renal failure are treated by peritoneal dialysis and most of the surgical and obstetric cases by haemodialysis using an arteriovenous shunt. As dialysis takes over the excretory function of the kidney, these ill patients no longer need to be starved. Attempts should be made to feed them 2500–3500 calories but their fluid intake as drinks should be restricted to 500 ml daily above their abnormal losses.

Dialysis techniques

Peritoneal dialysis (Fig. 33A)

The management of peritoneal dialysis is little more complicated than the management of an intravenous infusion régime. The patient does not need to be treated in a special dialysis unit or even an intensive care unit but often his general condition warrants this more specialized care.

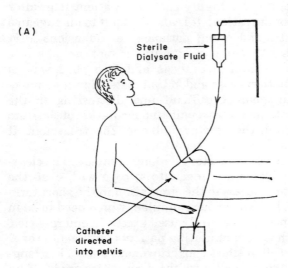

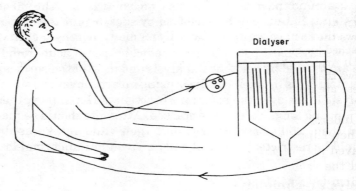

Fig. 33.
(A) Peritoneal dialysis. The plastic catheter is inserted into the pelvis under local anaesthesia (see Fig. 35). The direction of fluid in and out is controlled by clips on the 'Y' junction. The system is closed to prevent infection.

(B) Venovenous haemodialysis. A large-bore perforated catheter is inserted into the inferior vena cava via the long saphenous vein and takes blood to the dialyser. Blood is returned to any large peripheral vein. A blood pump is necessary on the exit side of the circuit.

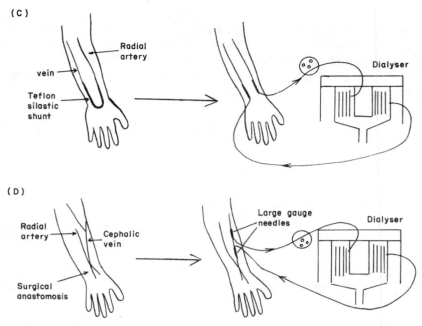

Fig. 33.
(C) Arteriovenous shunt haemodialysis. The diagram on the left shows the hook-up between dialysis. The silastic shunt is divided and attached to the inflow and outflow of the dialyser.
(D) Arteriovenous fistula haemodialysis. The diagram on the left shows the surgical anastomosis which leads to dilated forearm veins. These are needled to connect to the dialyser.

Under local anaesthesia a doctor inserts a peritoneal dialysis catheter into the peritoneal cavity through the lower half of the shaved abdominal wall. He avoids areas with laparotomy scars and the region of the inferior epigastric blood vessels. A point 3–6 cm below the umbilicus in the midline is a useful site. The catheter which is illustrated (Fig. 34) consists of a graduated nylon tube with multiple perforations and a trocar for its introduction. A metal disc is used to strap the catheter at the required depth and a flexible tube with a tap is used to connect it to the input and drainage bags. After anaesthetizing the skin and deeper tissues with 1% lignocaine a 3-mm skin incision is made. The trocar and catheter are inserted and when the catheter is in the peritoneal cavity the trocar is withdrawn. The catheter is then directed so that its tip is in the recto-vesical fossa of the pelvis. The depth of insertion is checked by the graduations on the tube and the metal disc is fitted. The excess tube is cut off. For chronic peritoneal dialysis a silastic catheter is used. This gives rise to less discomfort and peritonitis but may need an open operation and removal of the omentum for long-term success.

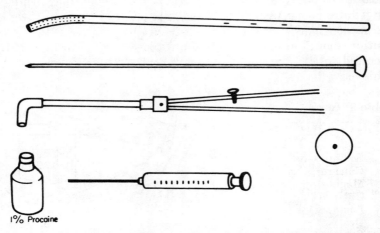

1% Procaine

Fig. 34. Peritoneal dialysis kit. From above down: plastic catheter with perforation and marks to gauge the depth of insertion, trocar, tubing to make the 'Y' hook-up, circular disc to fix catheter, local anaesthetic.

Dialysis can now commence. This can be done manually or by machine. Bags of dialysate fluid are warmed to 37°C in a water bath. A litre is run in under gravity from a height of about 1–1.5 m through a 'Y' connection. The fluid is allowed to equilibrate in the peritoneal cavity for twenty minutes. During this period diffusable substances (water, urea, sodium, potassium, acid, base) pass between the plasma and the fluid in the peritoneum in either direction depending on the concentration gradient present. The tap on the drainage tube to the bag beneath the bed is opened and the fluid is withdrawn. Accurate records of volumes in and out are charted. If the patient's condition is satisfactory 2-litre exchanges can be given with advantage. It is usual for each dialysis cycle to take 1 hour.

Machines are available to perform the in and out cycles automatically. These have a role in specialized units but the method described above is usually satisfactory in the ICU as patients of this type need close nursing supervision. In addition to measuring the patient's fluid balance, it is advantageous to check it by dialysing him on a weigh bed. Many units, however, do not have this equipment so that meticulous records of fluid volume exchanged are essential for safe management.

Samples of dialysis effluent should be cultured for bacteria and fungi daily. If organisms are grown or the effluent becomes turbid, the appropriate antibiotics can be added to the dialysate. Extreme caution should attend the use of antibiotics which are normally excreted in the urine (e.g. streptomycin) as toxic levels can be achieved with ease.

Table 2. Composition of peritoneal dialysis fluid.

	mmol/l	g/l	mmol/l	g/l
Sodium	140.4		140.40	
Calcium	3.6		3.6	
Magnesium	1.5		1.5	
Chloride	100.8		100.8	
Lactate	44.6		44.6	
Dextrose		13.6		63.6
Osmolarity*	364.37		642.91	

* Osmolarity of plasma 310–320

Two types of peritoneal dialysate fluid are available. They contain identical electrolyte concentrations but are rendered either slightly or strongly hypertonic by the addition of dextrose 1.5% or 7.0%. The latter allows the withdrawal of large quantities of water as the strong solution osmotically sucks water from the blood across the peritoneum. It is usual to use the strong solution for a proportion of the exchanges depending on the amount of water to be removed and on the circulatory effect on the patient. If used to excess these solutions bring about a massive contraction of the blood volume before it can be replaced by extracellular water. It is therefore essential to record the pulse and blood pressure regularly through dialysis, particularly when using the hypertonic solutions. The strongly hypertonic solutions also cause more abdominal pain than the weaker one. For this reason the fluid intake by mouth or drip needs to be restricted in patients on peritoneal dialysis.

On occasions peritoneal dialysis is unsatisfactory as the fluid volume collected falls short of that infused. This is usually due to loculation within the peritoneal cavity and can often be rectified by gentle repositioning of the catheter. If these measures and reinsertion of the catheter in another position fail, peritoneal dialysis may have to be abandoned in favour of haemodialysis.

It should be noted that the standard peritoneal dialysis fluid does not contain any potassium. This is because many patients requiring dialysis are hyperkalaemic. As potassium dialyses rapidly across a 6–7 mmol gradient, hypokalaemia can be produced after several 2-litre dialysate exchanges. It is, therefore, necessary to add 4 mmol/l to the dialysate as soon as acute hyperkalaemia has been treated (i.e. after the first 6–10 exchanges). The addition of 500 iu heparin to each litre of dialysis fluid facilitates the exchanges by preventing thrombus formation within the peritoneal cavity and subsequent blockage of the side holes in the catheter.

Once the acute imbalance has been rectified by peritoneal dialysis, using continuous 1-hour exchange cycles, the patients can be maintained by overnight dialysis for several weeks or even months if strict aseptic precautions are taken. However, in anything but the short term, haemodialysis is a more comfortable and safer treatment. Recently peritoneal dialysis has been used to manage patients with chronic renal failure. Continuous ambulatory peritoneal dialysis involves the patient infusing his own peritoneum about 5 times daily and allowing the fluid to drain 4–6 hours later. In the fit patient biochemical control and rehabilitation are excellent. The technique is particularly useful in very young and elderly patients who may have poor vessels for haemodialysis.

Haemodialysis

Haemodialysis involves taking the patient's blood from a convenient vessel and allowing it to pass across a semi-permeable membrane on the other side of which is the dialysate fluid. Four methods of access to the circulation are available.

1. Venovenous dialysis (Fig. 33B). This was the original method of haemodialysis. A large tube is placed in a central vein (usually the inferior vena cava) and blood is sucked out into the dialyser. After passage across the membrane the blood is returned to a large

peripheral vein through a cut-down cannula. These cannulae have to be reinserted for each dialysis or can be filled with heparin between dialyses. If they are left in for more than 7–14 days sepsis may occur around the cannulae and vena cava thrombosis is a common problem. This method is only suitable for short-term dialysis but has the advantage of requiring only two simple cut-down operations which is useful in very ill patients.

2. Arteriovenous dialysis and shunts. The finding that plastic tubes can be inserted into peripheral arteries and veins to make a short circuit for blood outside the body, revolutionized haemodialysis. Scribner in America devised the first of these tubes. Many modifications have been made since. We currently use two straight lengths of silastic tube joined by a Teflon connecter tube and inserted usually into the radial or posterior tibial artery and cephalic or long saphenous vein through Teflon tips (Fig. 33C). Some units prefer curved stepped shunts closer to the original design but we feel that the ease with which straight shunts can be declotted justified their use as a routine.

Between dialysis, blood short circuits from artery to vein through a silastic loop. The loop is divided to plug into the arterial and venous ends of the dialyser. The two major problems of shunts are clotting and sepsis. They also restrict the patient's activity as there is a risk of dislodging the shunt. In the acutely ill patient requiring intensive care it is important to avoid cannulating at least one limb for intravenous infusions, injections or blood sampling as the patient subsequently may need haemodialysis. We have seen several patients in whom it was difficult to establish satisfactory shunts because of previous damage to veins.

Arteriovenous shunts need careful management, especially in an ICU. The tubing should be fixed firmly to prevent dislodgement and pulling that will cause trauma to the intima of the vessel by the Teflon tip. The tube should be covered with dressings, leaving only a small segment visible to detect clotting. If the shunt is in the arm this should be elevated for 2–3 days after it has been inserted. If the shunt is in the leg the patient should not walk for ten days. Blood pressure should not be taken on a limb proximal to a shunt. Using full aseptic technique with gloves, blood samples can be obtained from the shunt with ease. This is particularly useful for arterial samples for PO_2, PCO_2 etc. On the other hand the shunt should not be used for the administration of drugs as this leads to thrombosis.

Clotting of an A-V shunt is caused either by damage to the
arterial or venous intima by trauma or infection or because of
hypotension. The latter is the most common cause encountered in
the ICU. It should be treated urgently. The cannulae can be declotted by gentle suction on the blood lines and gentle irrigation
through a catheter inserted up the line. Care should be taken not to
inject into a clotted shunt. The dangers of doing this through the
venous cannula are not very great and result only in a small
pulmonary embolus. The dangers on the arterial side can be disastrous with cerebral thrombus or air embolism. In the long term
anticoagulants may be useful to prevent recurrent clotting
episodes in shunts.

3. Arteriovenous fistulae. To overcome the problems of clotting
and sepsis with external plastic shunts, Cimino and Brescia
showed that adequate access to the circulation could be obtained
by percutaneous needling of the tortuous veins resulting from the
creation of an arteriovenous fistula. This method has little application in the treatment of acute renal failure as it is some weeks
before the veins are big enough to use. The intensive care nurses
will meet this type of patient in renal transplant units and when
patients on chronic dialysis enter intensive care units for other
reasons (Fig. 33D).

4. Single cannula dialysis. Recently modifications have been
made to dialysis circuits to allow dialysis to proceed using a needle
or cannula. Blood is withdrawn into the machine, dialysed and
then returned to the patient in a rhythmical three-phase cycle.

Haemodialysis machines

For the haemodialysis to take place two components are necessary—the dialyser itself, which is the true artificial kidney, and
the control unit which often provides the dialysate fluid and
monitors the dialysis. There are many different types of machine
and dialyser available and in a book of this type we only propose to
discuss two types of each.

The dialyser

The first practical clinical dialyser was used by Kolff during the
1939–1945 war. It consisted essentially of a sausage skin suspended in a bath of dialysate fluid. The patient's blood circulated

through the skin tube. The modern Kolff kidney is still available and used in some centres. It is a very efficient dialyser capable of high clearances. Its main problem is that it corrects the composition of the plasma too fast so that disequilibration may occur between the plasma and the extracellular fluid which can have undesirable effects on cardiovascular and central nervous function.

The Kiil dialyser which consists of flat sheets of cellophane mounted on a large flat frame and needs to be assembled for every or every other dialysis is becoming less used. This is because the modern disposable dialysers (coil, flat plate or capillary) are reasonably priced, reliable and less laborious to use. They can be re-used safely with very little labour thus reducing the unit cost of a haemodialysis even further.

Dialysate control systems

Two systems are available; the single patient proportionating system and the central dialysate supply system. The former allows patients to be dialysed in any part of the hospital or at home. The latter is only applicable in a large haemodialysis unit. Therefore the patient in an ICU is most likely to use a single-patient machine. Several makes are available. Each has its disadvantages and new models are being produced each year. To be generally applicable for ICU work the system should always be managed by specialized technicians, in the same way as ventilators. The ICU nurse should understand enough to make the hour-by-hour adjustments through a dialysis.

The single-patient units proportionately dilute concentrated dialysis solutions and monitor the concentration of the solution that the patient's blood is dialysed against, and the flow of blood. They continuously produce dialysate at 500 ml/min by diluting a concentrated dialysate with tap water using a special pump. The concentration of the dialysate is monitored electronically and if this varies outside preset limits, the dialyser is automatically bypassed. This makes it impossible to dialyse the patient against a grossly hypertonic or hypotonic solution. The temperature of the dialysate is controlled and indicated on a gauge. The pressure of the dialysate and its flow rate are controlled and monitored. A photoelectric cell detects small blood leaks and air bubbles and sounds audible and visual alarms and cuts out the blood and

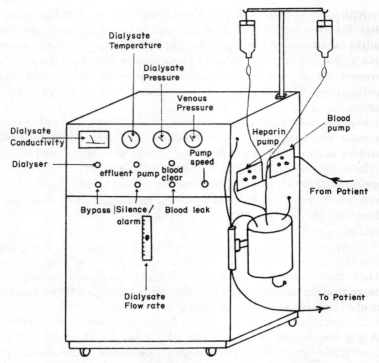

Fig. 35. Schematic representation of a kidney machine. The machine produces the dialysate fluid at the correct concentration (conductivity), temperature, pressure, flow rate and free from blood contamination. It also controls the rate of blood flow, its anticoagulation and ultrafiltration (venous pressure). The coil type dialyser is on a shelf on the right of the machine. The flat-bed Kiil dialyser would be free-standing. The alarm system is designed to be fail safe.

effluent pumps should a leak occur. The venous pressure of the return side of the blood line is measured and has automatic cut-outs which can be preset to allow ultrafiltration. Roller pumps of variable speed control the blood flow through the system and allow the administration of heparin to prevent clotting in the extracorporeal circuit. The heparin is fed into the arterial or input part of the circuit. This results in heparization of the patient during dialysis. The dose of heparin used with modern dialysis is small compared with the older models so that systematic bleeding is rare even in patients with recent trauma or operations. Regional heparinization is rarely required.

Although, unlike peritoneal dialysis, the dialysate for hae-modialysis machines does not need to be sterile, the dialysis circuit should be sterilized before use. This prevents the growth of bacteria and fungi in the circuit which on occasions appear to produce pyrogens which can pass through the membrane. Two methods of sterilization are in general use, chemical or heat. Chemical sterilization can be performed with formaldehyde or gluteraldehyde. This must be done manually and formalin causes problems because it is so pungent. Despite regular sterilization there is a build-up of dead microbial material in the dialysate circuit which can be seen through the plastic tubing. This needs to be changed at approximately monthly intervals. Heat sterilization machines have an automatic push-button sterilization cycle which is labour-saving. A 30-amp electricity supply is required for heat sterilizing machines.

The growth of organisms is largely dependent on the sugar content of the dialysate and can be reduced by using ultrafiltration rather than osmotic pressure to extract water from the patient. The composition of a standard dialysate fluid is given approximately in Table 3.

Table 3. Composition of a dialysate fluid in mmol/l.

Sodium	Na^+	132.0
Potassium	K^+	1.3
Magnesium	Mg^{++}	1.0
Calcium	Ca^{++}	3.0
Chloride	Cl^-	101.3
Lactate or Acetate		40.0
Dextrose	200 mg%	

Another potential hazard within kidney machines is blood contamination. Recent experiments have shown that micro-organisms can pass through the dialysis membranes into and out of the blood circuit. Also it has been shown that blood contamination over a radius of 3 m occurs during the connection of a patient to haemodialysis. The control buttons on the proportioning machine are particularly prone to contamination and should be carefully cleaned after each dialysis.

Connecting a patient to an artificial kidney

Cannulae will have been inserted into the circulation by the medical staff so that an outflow and an inflow to the patient are available. The dialyser is primed with dialysate. Only very rarely is it necessary to prime the extracorporeal circuit with blood even in children or the very sick as the volume of the circuit is small. In one system the dialyser only contains 25 ml of blood. The circuit is warmed to body temperature with saline and circulated to check for leaks. If all is well the blood pump is switched off and the blood lines are clamped and divided. The arterial line from the patient is joined to the inflow to the dialyser. If the dialyser has been primed with saline the patient is bled into the machine and the saline is allowed to run to waste until it is faintly pink. Then the venous side is connected. If a blood prime is used both lines are connected before any of the blood leaves the patient. The blood pump is started and dialysis is under way. The blood lines are fixed firmly and comfortably in position to allow the patient as much freedom of movement as possible and to allow the other nursing tasks to be performed. The newer plastic taps (Micropore) are of great help for this. The heparin pump is set to deliver approximately four drops per minute. The blood flow rate through the circuit can be checked by timing the progress of air injected into the arterial side of the circuit. Most dialysers require a rate of 150 ml/min to give satisfactory clearances. The rate of water removal can be adjusted by applying a gateclip to the venous line on the patient side of the bubble trap. Raising the venous pressure to 200 mmHg results in the removal of 100 ml water per hour. If more water needs to be removed the dextrose concentration of the dialysate can be increased to 2%

Discontinuing dialysis

Nowadays dialysis is usually a planned routine procedure and not a last-minute emergency. It is usual to plan a dialysis to run 4–6 hours depending on the machinery used. Dialysis can be discontinued at any time in an emergency by clamping the blood lines. This may need to be done if the membrane bursts or the extracorporeal circuit clots. It is usually necessary to start again with a blood prime for the machine as the patient's blood volume will be low. Sometimes when the membrane bursts it is possible to wash back most of the blood into the patient in the usual way.

At the end of a routine dialysis the dialyser contents are washed back into the patient by disconnecting the arterial line and infusing saline through this. There is a certain element of competition among dialysers and designers to salvage for the patient every red cell from the circuit by tipping the dialyser into different positions. 500–800 ml saline is usually used to wash back the dialyser blood. This is more important for patients on chronic dialysis than those with acute renal failure.

Further treatment of patients with renal failure

We have discussed some of the more technical aspects of correcting the fluid and electrolyte imbalance in anuric patients. Now let us consider what happens after the patient has been dialysed. One of three things will happen to an ICU patient who has renal failure. He may make a complete recovery from his illness and his renal failure. He may recover from his illness and be left with irreparably damaged kidneys or he may die from his illness. The second alternative is uncommon. It is usually necessary to dialyse the patient for 2–3 weeks before recovery occurs but occasionally dialysis for 3–4 months is necessary before the kidneys make a virtually full recovery. As the catabolic rate of most ICU patients is high, dialysis on alternate days is usually necessary to maintain reasonable serum chemistry. This should be checked daily (Na^+, K^+, urea). Any acid-base imbalance will be rapidly corrected by dialysis so regular checks are not necessary unless there is some other indication. When anuria has developed, any urethral catheter should normally be removed to prevent infection. There is little danger of failing to detect the recovery phase from anuria as the daily urine volume will rise over 2–3 days from under 400 ml to 2000 ml or more. A very large diuresis usually means that the patient was overhydrated in the anuric phase. Dialysis can usually be discontinued in a patient with acute renal failure when the urine volume has been over 1000 ml for 2 days. A careful check on the urine chemistry is necessary to monitor the improvement in urea and creatinine clearance and to detect the occasional excessive sodium diuresis. The fluid intake during the diuretic phase should match the previous days urine volume. There is little evidence to suggest that an episode of acute renal failure has a deleterious effect on the long-term function of the kidney. One of our patients was anuric for 14 weeks following a hypotensive episode after cholecystectomy. Twelve months later his renal function, as judged by creatinine clearance and urinalysis, was normal.

Occasionally ICU patients will survive with inadequate renal function. One of our first transplant patients presented to our ICU with acute renal and respiratory failure associated with pregnancy. The need for prolonged ventilation and intravenous fluid and drug administration resulted in thrombosis of many of her peripheral veins. This made her maintenance on a long-term dialysis difficult. She received a cadaveric renal transplant a year later and now has normal renal function more than a decade later.

Renal transplantation

Like the patient just described, more and more patients with irreversible acute or chronic renal failure are being submitted for a renal transplant. The widespread clinical application of this technique is very greatly facilitated by dialysis. By this means the general health of patients with renal failure can be improved so that they are better able to withstand the transplant operation and the post-operative immunosuppressive therapy. It is unlikely that patients on chronic dialysis will enter intensive care units unless some major catastrophe occurs. For example, a weekend of gross dietary and fluid indiscretion will, by increasing the water, salt and potassium intake, send a patient into left ventricular failure and hyperkalaemia. On occasions such patients will need intermittent positive pressure ventilation and cardiac monitoring until dialysis can remove the water and salt load and reduce the serum potassium.

Although the operation of renal transplantation is routine in most transplant centres and most patients cause no anxieties at that time, they are in a vulnerable state. If anything goes wrong you are usually faced with a string of life-threatening consequences.

It is now accepted that one should transplant the patient with the best tissue-type-matched kidney. As many patients have to wait many months for a kidney to become available, they may just be due for a dialysis when the kidney arrives. They will at that time be relatively overhydrated, hyperkalaemic and uraemic. They are also chronically anaemic. We accept a patient as 'fit' for transplant if his haemoglobin is above 5 g %, potassium under 6.2 mmol, urea under 35 mmol/l and he has no clinical signs of overhydration (peripheral or pulmonary oedema) or he has gained no more than 2 kg body weight since the last dialysis.

Post-operatively the patients must be carefully observed. They do not become cyanosed at this level of haemoglobin concentration even if their ventilatory function is very depressed. We usually administer 30% oxygen through a face mask for 24 hours post-operatively. It is rarely necessary to dialyse a patient post transplant as with kidneys from live donors or heart beating cadavers, immediate function is the norm.

Relationship between ICU and dialysis unit

It is becoming increasingly clear that the patients' needs in intensive care units and dialysis units are very similar. To be able to function smoothly there is much to be said for the nursing and medical training in these units to be integrated. In our hospital group an attempt is made to rotate nursing and medical staff between the two, although administratively they are separate.

Other organ transplants

The addition of immunosuppressive treatment and the coincident depression of resistance to infection of a patient under intensive care, calls for the isolation of the patient from exogenous infection. Recently, renal transplant patients have received more conservative doses of immunosuppressive drugs as it is realized that it is safer to allow the graft to be rejected than to push the drugs to the limit. The artificial kidney makes this possible.

When we consider liver, lung or heart transplants there is little choice because when the graft is rejected there is seldom the chance of a second transplant. Leukopenic patients with functioning, albeit poorly, grafts are commonplace. Reversed barrier intensive nursing is the present-day answer. It is unsatisfactory because the patient often succumbs to an endogenous infection with an organism which is usually a harmless passenger in the patient's bowel or respiratory tract. The ultimate answer will be more specific immunosuppression, abolishing the response to the graft but leaving the body's defences against infection unimpaired.

Viral hepatitis

Long incubation viral or serum hepatitis is common in the patients and staff of dialysis and transplant units. The presence of the virus is detected by a serological test (HBsAg). The severity of the disease caused by this virus varies from one that is highly lethal to one that causes only mild biochemical upsets of transaminase and bilirubin.

The disease probably enters a dialysis unit in the first place in an infected bag of blood (1 in 1000 blood donors is HBsAg positive). Patients on dialysis or after transplantation have a suppressed immune system and become chronic carriers of the virus. The infection is transmitted to other patients by blood contamination of the kidney machine (particularly through the venous pressure manometer) and to the staff and their relatives by accidental inoculation of blood by needles, by splashing into the eye or by passage from the fingers to the mouth. One small drop of serum contains many infective doses of virus. Recently it has been shown that the urine of HBsAg positive patients is also infective.

This infection can be prevented by:

1. Using HBsAg negative blood in renal units
2. Using only HBsAg negative organ donors
3. Excluding HBsAg positive staff and patients from the unit

Further, protective gowns, gloves and masks should be used in all dealings with the blood of dialysis patients (venepuncture, declotting shunts etc.). If an infected patient is detected in the unit, he should be isolated immediately and either transferred to home dialysis, to a special isolation dialysis unit or receive a kidney transplant. Only by meticulous care can the risks of this and other as yet undescribed infections be limited in renal units. In general, blood should be regarded as 'dirty' fluid in the same way as faeces. If a member of the staff or any other person becomes contaminated by blood from an HBsAg positive person there is evidence of the benefit from the administration of specific gammaglobulin. This must be given as soon as possible after the inoculation. There is recent evidence that a surgeon may contract the disease by operating on a known carrier despite full precautions. He may also infect another patient during the postdromal phase of the clinical disease. Another surgeon infected a series of patients. He was found to be an asymptomatic carrier of HBsAg. These examples support a policy of regular screening in a renal unit.

It is usual to separate patients with acute renal failure, where the carriage of hepatitis is usually unknown, from chronic renal failure patients who have been thoroughly screened before entry to the unit.

Chapter 8
Care of the Unconscious Patient

The unconscious patient poses problems in management which result mainly from the lack of information he is able to feed back to his doctors and nurses and from the loss in his own normal protective mechanisms. For example the unconscious patient may not complain of pain which may be a useful guide to some pathological process or he may not be able adequately to separate his food and air passages.

Scope of the problem

It is common to find patients unconscious from many causes in intensive care units. The type of the unconsciousness seen will depend on the role of the unit. A unit in a hospital with a busy accident department will have a high percentage of patients with head injuries whereas in other units the most common diagnosis may be drug overdose or subarachnoid haemorrhage. Despite the multiplicity of causes, the general management of the unconscious patient varies little.

It is, however, important to arrive at a diagnosis of the cause of the unconscious state at the earliest opportunity because urgent treatment may be necessary to prevent permanent brain damage. For example, a young epileptic lady was taken to the emergency department following a 999 call. Earlier that afternoon she had collected a prescription for barbiturates and tranquillizers from her family doctor. She collapsed in the doorway of the butcher's shop, apparently tripping on the step. In her handbag were found empty tablet bottles. On admission she was deeply unconscious, failing to respond to any stimulus and gradually her breathing became inadequate. She was intubated and was transferred to the ICU on a ventilator. The diagnosis lay between post-convulsional state, drug overdose, head injury or a combination. A skull X-ray did not reveal a fracture and physical examination failed to reveal any abnormality. A massive barbiturate overdose was the most likely diagnosis. Blood was sent for examination and preparations were made to dialyse the patient. No barbiturate was detected in the blood. Re-examination of the patient revealed a small bruise on the scalp. Echo-encephalography revealed a gross midline shift of the brain and autopsy confirmed an acute subdural haematoma. This patient illustrates the speed at which it is necessary to work to diagnose and treat the unconscious patient. The clinician looking after an unconscious patient must aim to get his priorities right, he must be made aware of a life-threatening sign by those in minute-to-minute care of his patient. This responsibility rests very firmly on the nurse in the ICU. This task is a tremendous challenge to her.

In addition to the diagnosis and the specific treatment the most usual problems with the unconscious patient are concerned with maintaining adequate ventilation, an adequate circulation, fluid, electrolyte and food intake and getting rid of the excreta.

Nursing observations

A patient who loses normal consciousness from whatever cause, goes through the same stages, albeit at different rates. These have been called levels of consciousness and are similar to the stages of anaesthia. Several classifications have been devised but the levels displayed in Table 4 have been found very useful.

Table 4. A useful classification of the levels of consciousness.

Conscious level	Reflexes	Pupils
1. Normal	Normal	react to light and accommodation
2. Confused	Normal	as level 1
3. Reacts to simple commands	Normal	may be irregular
4. Reacts purposefully to pain	Vary	as level 3
5. Reacts non-purposefully to pain	Vary	as level 3
6. No response to pain	None	fixed dilated

Level 1 is normal consciousness and this may or may not be accompanied by focal signs. These may present as a derangement of movement or reflexes. Level 6 is one stage above death and is frequently associated with inadequate ventilation, a failing circulation and falling body temperature. If maintained for some hours it may indicate irrecoverable cerebral damage (Fig. 36).

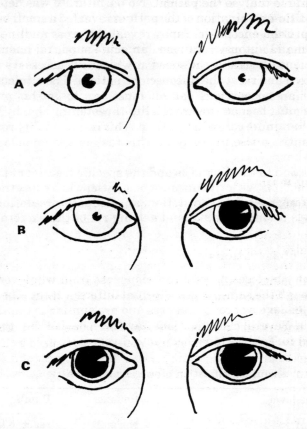

Fig. 36. Pupil changes after head injury. (A) Increase in intracranial pressure has produced constriction of the left pupil; (B) later the left pupil is paralysed and widely dilated and the right pupil is now constricted; (C) gross elevation of intracranial pressure has produced bilateral fixed dilated pupils.

It is important to observe and record the level of consciousness regularly so that the progress of the patient can be assessed. This is best done by the nurse as she can observe fluctuation of response which may be extremely helpful diagnostic signs. This is particularly true when patients require artificial ventilation and may be receiving drugs which abolish spontaneous respiration and other movements. The observations should be recorded on a flow chart using a standard nomenclature so that there is conformity between nurses of successive shifts.

In addition to the conscious level, pulse rate, blood pressure and temperature should be recorded regularly. A slowing pulse rate and rising blood pressure may indicate increasing intracranial pressure, the converse may indicate bleeding. It is often more accurate to record the rectal rather than the oral temperature. A high temperature may be a sign of intercranial haemorrhage. On the other hand, it may indicate a respiratory infection. Hypothermia in patients on a ventilator, if progressive, is often a sign of irreversible cerebral damage.

Nursing management

Very careful attention must be paid to the general care of the unconscious patient as he is very prone to decubitus ulceration if he is not turned regularly and his pressure areas treated. Care should also be taken not to put his limbs through abnormal movements as these can result in injuries such as dislocated shoulder. The limb joints should be put through their full range of normal movement to encourage the circulation to the limb and prevent joint stiffness.

It is important to make certain that none of the apparatus attached to the patient can cause injury. For example a clamp on a drainage tube can very easily stick into the patient's skin and cause an ulcer. Patients can be burned due to a short circuit through any metal connector but nowadays plastic connectors avoid this.

Care must also be taken to protect the patients' eyes from damage. When unconscious, the eyes are insensitive so that foreign bodies can impinge on the corneal surface and cause ulceration. If the eyes are closed this risk is minimized and the cornea is protected from damage from desiccation by exposure. Micropore tape is useful to tape the lids closed. Tulle gras pads or liquid paraffin eyedrops are useful to prevent desiccation which leads to corneal ulceration.

The liberal use of unmedicated talcum powder, sheepskin rugs, ripple mattresses and beds that can be tipped in either direction greatly facilitate the general nursing of the patient. The temperature of the ICU should be maintained about 70°F so that the minimum of bedclothes is required as these interfere with the minute-to-minute care and observation of the patient.

The management of the ventilatory function of the unconscious patient has been fully discussed in Chapters 4 and 5. It is sufficient to remind the nurse that the unconscious patient is unable to tell us he is dyspnoeic. If he is restless but unconscious it is difficult to judge the adequacy of ventilation. You should look for signs of airway obstruction and cyanosis and if there is any doubt the arterial PO_2 and PCO_2, pH and standard HCO_3 should be estimated. It may be necessary to depress the level of consciousness of the overactive disorientated patient with respiratory insufficiency so that he may be intubated and ventilated. This is one reason why the serial recordings of the level of consciousness are so important.

Patients with any depression of conscious level below minor disorientation cannot take oral fluids or food without a severe risk of aspiration into the tracheobronchial tree. If unconsciousness lasts more than a day it is essential to institute fluid administration and feeding. When there is no abdominal pathology this is best done by an indwelling nasogastric tube. Through this, an adequate intake of fluids and food can be given (Chapter 6). If there is abdominal pathology the intravenous route must be used for fluid and electrolyte therapy. If the unconscious state is expected to last for more than 2–3 days a catheter should be placed in a central vein or vena cava for parenteral feeding. Care must be taken to protect the site of an intravenous cannula to reduce the risks of infection. In the restless patient and during nursing procedures, care must be taken to prevent the cannula being displaced.

The nursing of the unconscious patient is facilitated by the presence of an indwelling urethral catheter. A full bladder causes excessive restlessness and repeated incontinence causes the decubitus skin to become soggy. The modern Foley or Gibbon catheters can be inserted into most patients and give adequate bladder drainage with a tolerably low rate of urinary tract infection. Systemic antibiotics should be given for clinical urinary infections as directed by the bacterial sensitivities. Some units use daily Noxyflex installations as a prophylaxis but there is no conclusive evidence of their efficacy.

If the patient has oliguric renal failure there are good reasons to remove the urinary catheter even in the unconscious patient. A diuresis will be heralded by a flood of urine which may be the indication for recatherization if unconsciousness persists (Chapter 7).

Let us now consider the more specific management of some of the common causes of unconsciousness seen in the ICU.

Head injuries

With the increase in high speed road traffic accidents, head injuries are increasingly common. The mortality rate from these injuries is high but can be reduced by better treatment. We need to consider three types of head injury.

Simple concussion

The patient who has sustained trauma to the head with probable loss of consciousness which was transient. There may or may not be a fractured skull. These patients need to be admitted for observation to make sure that there is no subsequent loss of consciousness indicating haemorrhage within the skull (middle meningeal artery, extra dural haemorrhage or subdural haemorrhage) which will require urgent operation.

Patients with simple concussion may require surgical treatment such as elevation of a depressed fracture but commonly only need bed rest and observation for 24–72 hours. It is a tragedy if a patient dies as a result of this type of injury. Most deaths can be prevented by very careful observation and swift action as soon as any deterioration occurs. Although these patients should be nursed in intensive care units there is often insufficient room and they are 'observed' in the general ward. This is very much less satisfactory as they may well appear to be the fittest patients on the ward and are often thought to be hardly worth a bed. Nevertheless about 1 in 1000 may deteriorate over a very short period and die from brain compression.

Sustained unconsciousness

The second group of patients are those who were rendered unconscious by the injury and have not regained consciousness. They may or may not have adequate spontaneous breathing. The precise pathology within the skull is at first unknown but usually physical examination aided by such measures as X-rays, ultrasound, computerized tomography or arteriography have failed to reveal evidence of local damage. Were they to have done so this may have been an indication for exploratory burr holes as a means of decompressing the brain.

These patients are usually nursed in the ICU where due attention to the recordings previously outlined can be given. The adequacy of ventilation is checked frequently and if recovery does not take place during the first 24 hours fluid replacement and feeding are instituted. Some surgeons believe that the cerebral state after head injuries can be improved by attempting to shrink the brain by the administration of hypertonic substances intravenously. Urea and dextrose can be used. The raised osmolarity of the serum drains fluid out from the brain into the blood. There is no conclusive evidence that these measures are effective. Some units now monitor intracranial pressure through an indwelling cannula and treat sustained rises in pressure aggressively. Others cause fluid depletion by giving mannitol or frusemide to cause a diuresis. Again no conclusive benefit has been found. Care should be taken not to take the dehydration procedures too far as they can render the patient uraemic. We have had occasion to speed the recovery of a patient unconscious from a head injury who had been given the 'drying out' regime. He was offered to us as a potential kidney donor. As he was severely oliguric we suggested that we were not interested until his kidneys had been shown to work. He was rehydrated and made a prompt recovery.

Multiple injuries

The third group of head-injury patients are those in whom the head injury is only one of several injuries. The head injury makes the assessment of the other injuries difficult and often the skills of the veterinary surgeon must be relied upon. Likewise the other injuries may make the severity of the head injury difficult to judge and may obscure focal signs. For example, recently we took over the care of a 15-year-old girl pedestrian who had been hit by a car in the left loin. On arrival at the accident department she was in respiratory distress and profoundly hypotensive. She appeared to be able to move her arms but not her legs. There were conflicting observations of her state of consciousness. As a life-saving measure she was intubated, ventilated and transfused. At operation a few hours later a left nephrectomy and splenectomy were performed to stop uncontrolled bleeding. A large left haemothorax was evacuated. The compound tibial fracture was immobilized in plaster of Paris and she was nursed on her back because of an extensive fracture dislocation of the spine at L 2–3 level. Despite 20 units of blood she was hypotensive for some hours and developed acute tubular necrosis of the remaining right kidney. Surprisingly she was alive 2 days later and was transferred to our ICU for haemodialysis and further treatment. During the ensuing month her renal function improved and she was weaned from the ventilator. Unfortunately her cerebral function was very slow to recover. At autopsy 6 weeks later both frontal and temporal lobes of the brain were necrotic.

In her initial treatment this young girl posed great problems in diagnosis, particularly the extent of the head injury. Had the brain damage not been so severe, this girl was well worth saving. As it was there was no way of forecasting this earlier. It is in the treatment of this type of patient that the wits of all the experts, medical, nursing and technical, are tested to the limit. It is this that makes the work so stimulating.

Poisonings and overdoses

Many poisonous substances taken by accident or as a suicide attempt render the patient unconscious. The commonest type of patient requiring treatment is the one who is unconscious from aspirin, barbiturate or other sedative or tranquillizer overdose and now less commonly coal gas poisoning. The initial treatment of these patients is performed in the emergency department before admission to the ICU. This is immediate attention to respiratory function and methods to prevent absorption of the drug (e.g. stomach lavage) or specific drug antagonists (e.g. nalorphine, Megimide). Mild cases of drug overdose will probably not be admitted to the ICU which will be reserved for those who have a diminished level of consciousness from the drug.

The principle of treatment once the patient is in hospital is to remove the drug from the system in the most expeditious way and to maintain the patient's ventilation and circulation during this time. Drugs may be eliminated by the respiratory tract (coal gas, paraldehyde etc.) or by the kidneys (barbiturate, aspirin, amphetamine etc.) with or without prior detoxification in the liver. It is not the role of the nurse to decide on the method of treatment but in order to carry out the treatment she is advised to be acquainted with some of the effects of the common poisons and especially some of the new ones. Every year more chemicals are available and so the range of toxic actions increases continuously. This has lead to the establishment of regional centres where advice may be sought at any time on all types of poisoning.

In general terms, drugs which are taken in overdose fall into two groups—those which kill by respiratory depression and those which do not primarily depress the breathing but which disturb either the metabolism of the body or the cardiovascular system.

The largest number of overdose cases fall into the first category since they take sleeping tablets, tranquillizers and antidepressants, all of which kill primarily by respiratory depression. With these drugs it would be fair to say that provided that adequate mechanical ventilation can be maintained, the vast proportion of patients will recover even if nothing else is done in the way of management.

As regards the second group, however—especially aspirin— careful management of the patient's biochemical state, blood pressure and cardiac arrhythmia, if present, is essential even though mechanical ventilation is not required.

Coal gas

Carbon monoxide or coal gas combines with haemoglobin in the red cells to the exclusion of oxygen. It renders the patient grossly hypoxic although he becomes bright red (Carboxyhaemoglobin is redder than oxyhaemoglobin.) The carbon monoxide is excreted through the lungs and is displaced from haemoglobin by high concentrations of oxygen. The treatment is therefore to increase the oxygen concentration in the inspired air. Unless this is started promptly and sustained, anoxic brain damage will result with permanent impairment of the intellect or death.

Coal gas poisoning is becoming less common with the introduction, in town supplies, of natural gas which is non-toxic.

Barbiturate

Every type of barbiturate has been taken in overdose. The result is largely dose dependent. Barbiturates reduce cerebral activity progressively by blunting the higher intellectual functions first and the medullary function last. Barbiturates are detoxicated by the liver and excreted by the kidneys. This excretion is aided by a high urine flow. Mechanical ventilation is often essential. Haemodialysis has a role in patients with very high serum barbiturate levels but these are not common.

Aspirin

This poison is freely available without prescription. In addition to producing unconsciousness it is an acid and reduces the blood pH very profoundly by overcoming the buffering systems of the blood. This often results in very rapid breathing. In addition to the previously described measures a forced diuresis with an alkaline solution such as lactate or bicarbonate is beneficial. Haemodialysis removes salicylate but is rarely needed.

Stimulants

Amphetamine overdose is characterized by a very fast pulse rate and may mimic thyrotoxicosis. The drug is detected in the urine by the laboratory. It is usually necessary to sedate the patient in order to control the tachycardia and this may cause unconsciousness. Caution should be exercised as many of these patients have not simply taken a single drug as many amphetamine capsules also contain barbiturates or tranquillizers.

Tranquillizers and other sedatives

Over the past decade, a very large range of drugs has been introduced to treat mild and severe emotion problems. These substances taken in excess all lead to unconsciousness. During the recovery from unconsciousness, patients who have imbibed these may present with a bizarre range of neurological signs and symptoms. For example a patient who was being treated with chlorpromazine and who took some Mandrax tablets was found deeply unconscious without any response to pain or other stimuli. During the recovery phase she had a total aphasia for 3 days suggesting focal neurological damage. This resolved over the next 24 hours.

Opiates

Drug addiction is increasingly common, particularly in young persons. It is often possible to suspect the problem from the telltale injection marks. Opiates cause very marked respiratory depression and anoxia.

Alcohol

The drunkard often gets no further than the emergency department but he may be admitted to the ICU if he lapses into a coma. When presented with a patient who smells of drink, always be careful as he may have some underlying condition which is hidden by the alcohol and may require urgent treatment. Only recently there was a coroner's case of a man sent away from an emergency department as drunk only to die the next day of his head injury.

Overventilation

Overventilation will lead to a reduction in carbon dioxide levels in the blood, which in turn, causes constriction of the cerebral vessels. The effect may vary from a dreamy state to unconsciousness. Improvement is produced by adjusting the ventilator or increasing the dead space.

Rare causes

Recently the substance paraquat, a weedkiller, has been responsible for several cases of poisoning. It appears to be a particularly insidious and lethal poison. Symptoms do not come on for some days but when they do death follows. The patient develops a proliferative lung condition which causes breathlessness and anoxia. Lung transplantation has been attempted to overcome this condition but the new lung was destroyed by the residual poison.

Recently a case of physostigmine poisoning was admitted to our unit. This was taken deliberately by a graduate research worker. Prolonged ventilator treatment, nasogastric feeding and good ICU nursing enabled the patient to be maintained while he metabolized and excreted the drug.

Patients affected by the complex toxins of some infections such as tetanus, require ICU treatment. With tetanus the patient has convulsive episodes which lead to respiratory failure and death. In this case the patients must be sedated, paralysed and ventilated, until the convulsions wear off. They often become hyperpyrexial and must be cooled by fans and ice.

Anoxic unconsciousness

When the ICU is associated with a trauma and cardiothoracic surgical unit surgical unit cases of anoxic unconsciousness, often associated with low cardiac output states are common. These patients may also be suffering from cerebral air embolism or cerebral fat embolism.

The usual story is that the patient fails to wake up promptly after injury or surgery and has little or no localizing signs. The vital functions of respiration, blood pressure and temperature control may or may not be preserved. It is necessary to maintain the patient with or without ventilator assistance so that a diagnosis can be made. This usually takes two to three days. If the anoxic period causes cerebral oedema which leads to unconsciousness this usually recovers within this period. If unconsciousness is more prolonged the condition is usually irreversible.

Brain death

When an unconscious patient requires ventilation treatment there are three possible outcomes:

1. The patient may return to complete normality
2. The patient may have a permanent cerebral defect and if this is severe may result in a vegetative state
3. The patient may be or become brain dead

The possibility of complete recovery or a minimal residual defect is what is desired. A vegetative state is what is feared. Death is sometimes inevitable.

During the past decade the management of these severely ill patients has been better understood and guidelines have been agreed by the Conference of the Royal Colleges and Faculties of the United Kingdom on the criteria for the diagnosis of brain death.

Criteria for diagnosing brain death (to be carried out separately
by two doctors)

1. Nature of irremediable structural brain damage
2. Apnoeic coma, not due to
   a. depressant drugs
   b. neuromuscular blocking (relaxant) drugs
   c. hypothermia
   d. metabolic or endocrine disturbances
3. Pupils both fixed to light
4. Corneal reflex absent
5. No eye movements with cold caloric test
6. No cranial nerve motor responses
7. No gag reflex
8. No respiratory movements on disconnection from ventilator
   ($PaCO_2$ to rise above 50 mmHg)

It will be noted that advances have been made in the diagnosis of
death since the previous edition of this book. The falling blood
pressure and temperature occur as late signs of brain stem failure.
A flat electroencephalogram is a misleading test as a flat trace
does not indicate brain death neither does an active one mean that
brain stem death has not occurred. Isotope or CT scanning or
arteriography have not been found to add to the accuracy of the
clinical diagnosis.

Once the diagnosis of brain death has been made it has been
agreed that the patient is dead. This allows precise timing of death
which may have important legal implications in accident victims
where more than one member of a family may be involved. The
moment of cessation of artificial ventilation in no way determines
the moment of death neither is it related to the cessation of cardiac
activity in a brain-dead patient. This view is supported by the
experience of a series of patients diagnosed as being brain dead in
whom the ventilator was not discontinued. All had a spontaneous
cardiac arrest within 25 hours of the diagnosis of brain death.

There is an extensive education programme in the diagnosis of
death aimed at professional and lay audiences. As a result there is
a wide acceptance of brain death by the public. This is supported by
the lack of antagonistic response to the public statements by the
Conference of the Royal Colleges and Faculties. Despite this, need-
less to say, great tact and sympathy is necessary when dealing

with the relatives of these patients. It is sometimes a relief to the relatives to know that death has occurred despite everything that has been done to try to save life.

Cadaveric transplantation

Sometimes benefit for others can come from such a disaster. There is an increasing need for organs for transplantation, in particular for kidneys and corneas but in some centres the liver, pancreas and heart are also required. Publicity about the beneficial effects of organ transplantation has been aided by the provision of kidney donor cards (Fig. 37). These indicate the views of the person concerning cadaveric donation.

The legal basis of cadaveric transplantation is covered by the *Human Tissue Act 1961* which is a permissive law allowing removal of tissues and organs unless there is objection. A code of practice has been formulated by the DHSS in the United Kingdom to facilitate the supply of organs and especially kidneys.

1. Permission to go ahead with organ removal must be given by a person(s) delegated to do so by the person in possession of the body (AHA).
2. This permission can be given if the person in his lifetime expressed a lack of objection to donation.
3. If the views of the person are unknown such enquiries as are practical must be made to ascertain a lack of objection from the relatives.
4. If the case would normally be reported to the Coroner, his lack of objection must be obtained. In some areas Coroners have given blanket consent for certain types of case but other Coroners require to know each case as it presents. It is important to know the views of the local Coroner dealing with cases in your ICU.
5. Brain death, that is death, should be diagnosed by two independent doctors not connected with the transplant team, one of whom should be the consultant treating the patient and one other doctor. This diagnosis with its time should be recorded in the case records (Fig. 38).
6. The local transplant team should be notified at an early stage of any possible potential donor so that if the organs are available they can make best use of them.
7. It is legal and ethical to perform tests such as tissue typing

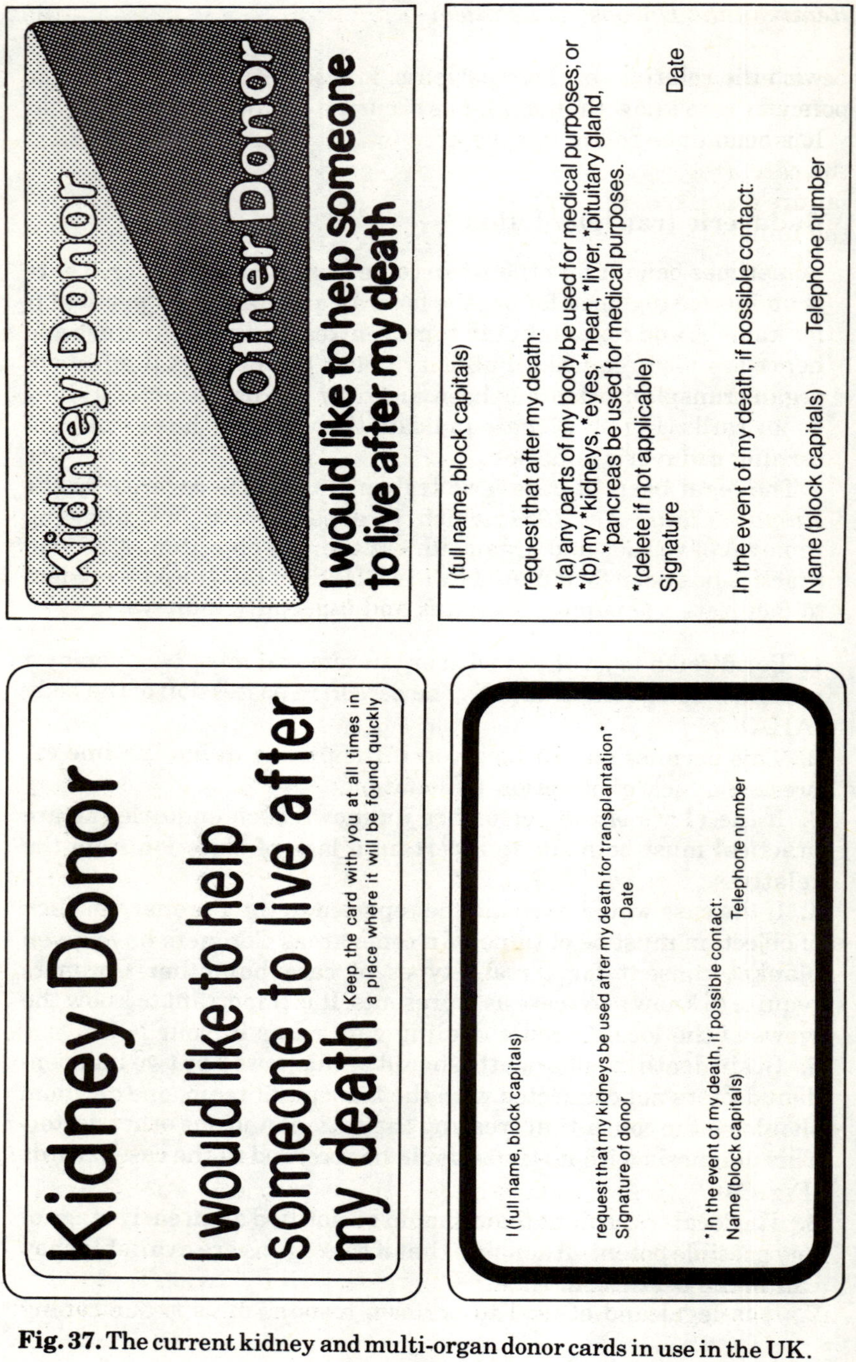

Fig. 37. The current kidney and multi-organ donor cards in use in the UK.

TRANSPLANTATION CHECKLIST   APPENDIX 3

Name of patient _____ Age _____

Home address _____

Hospital number _____

Name and address of next-of-kin _____

_____

Address of local transplant team _____

_____ Tel. _____

PART A.   ADMINISTRATIVE AND LEGAL MEASURES
Code of Practice

Paragraph

27	I DIAGNOSIS OF DEATH (See Part B for checklist of criteria for diagnosing brain death)
	Date and time diagnosis made _____
28	Names and status of doctors carrying out diagnosis
	1. _____
	2. _____
8	II IF A REQUEST HAD BEEN MADE FOR REMOVAL OF ORGANS AFTER DEATH FOR TRANSPLANTATION SPECIFY NATURE OF REQUEST, AND WHICH ORGANS
	Has patient requested removal of organs? if so, how _____
	Organs specified _____
8	Views of relatives if known _____ (Provided this is not a Coroner's or Procurator Fiscal's case authorization may now be given)
9	III IF THERE WAS NO EVIDENCE THAT A PATIENT HAD REQUESTED THE REMOVAL OF HIS ORGANS SPECIFY ENQUIRES MADE
12	Name and status of person(s) making enquiries _____
9, 10	Name and relationship of person(s) approached (i.e. parent, spouse, friend, cohabitee etc) _____
12	Date and nature (i.e. personal/telephone) and outcome of interview(s)

Fig. 38. Suggested documentation for organ donations.

Guidelines

Paragraph

14	If such reasonable enquiries as may be practicable were made, but views could not be obtained, state reasons _____ _____ _____ _____ (Provided this is not a Coroner's/Procurator Fiscal's case authorization may now be given if there is no reason to believe that there is a relevant objection)
17–19	**IV IF CASE IS ONE NORMALLY TO BE REPORTED TO CORONER/ PROCURATOR FISCAL HIS CONSENT TO REMOVAL OF ORGANS MUST BE OBTAINED**
20	Name and status of person approaching Coroner/Procurator Fiscal _____
20	Organs specified for removal _____ Date and time consent given _____ If consent withheld, state reasons _____ (Individual hospitals are advised to add a passage here setting out local Coroner's/Procurator Fiscal's practice)
	AUTHORIZATION Date and time authorization given _____ How given ('phone, orally, etc) _____ Signature of person to whom authorization communicated _____ Name of designated person _____
34	**V REMOVAL OF ORGANS** Name of doctor carrying out removal _____
34	Is doctor removing organs satisfied 1. by personal examination of the body that the patient is dead ▢ 2. where necessary, Coroner has given consent/ Procurator Fiscal has not objected ▢
33	Time organs removed _____ Any relevant pathology _____ _____ _____

Fig. 38. cont.

PART B.   CRITERIA FOR DIAGNOSING BRAIN DEATH
(to be carried out separately by 2 doctors)

Code of Practice

Paragraph

28	Nature of irremediable structural brain damage		
	Apnoeic coma, <u>not</u> due to:	Dr A	Dr B
	depressant drugs		
	neuromuscular blocking (relaxant) drugs		
	hypothermia		
	metabolic or endocrine disturbances		
	Pupils both fixed to light		
	Corneal reflex absent		
	No eye movements with cold caloric test		
	No cranial nerve motor reflexes		
	No gag reflex		
	No respiratory movements on disconnection (PaCO$_2$ to rise above 50 mmHg)		

NAME _____

STATUS _____

SIGNATURE _____

TIME _____

DATE _____

*Based on the detailed criteria drawn up by the Conference of Royal Colleges in 1976 (*Lancet* 1976, ii, 1069; *BMJ* 1976, ii, 1187)

Fig. 38. cont.

before death but no tests or investigations should be performed on a patient before death where these are only for the purposes of transplantation and are not in any way for the benefit of the dying patient.

8. After death has been diagnosed it is legal and ethical to perform tests and give treatment to the corpse for the benefit of the organ transplant. Such treatment often includes ventilation, hydration and drug treatment but in most circumstances should not be continued for more than 12 hours after death has been diagnosed.

9. The operative removal of organs from a corpse should be performed under normal surgical operating conditions. There are no legal or ethical objections to this being performed while ventilation and a normal circulation continues in a corpse after death has been diagnosed. Such an approach is essential for liver and heart transplantation and is preferred in kidney transplantation as this gives the best chance of immediate graft function.

10. Increasingly the relatives of the seriously ill volunteer the use of organs for transplantation and any request should be received sympathetically. It is often made to the nurse as she has the closest contact with the patient and relatives. Sometimes a patient is unsuitable as a donor for some organs (for example if there has been previous neoplasia, if there is gross sepsis or if there is impaired function of the organ concerned). In these cases it is good practice to explain carefully to the relatives the reasons why the organs are not wanted.

11. It is important to maintain the anonymity of the donor and recipients and to avoid publicity in the media

12. A full record of the donation should be recorded and be retained in a readily identifiable way in the patients case records. A suitable format has been suggested by the DHSS Working Party on transplantation (Fig. 38). For further details the reader is referred to the Working Party's Guidelines which are distributed to all UK ICUs 1980.

When organs have been offered for transplantation the local transplant team should be contacted. They have a central organization (UK Transplant) which links all the transplant units in the UK and advises as to the most suitable recipient for the organs. There are links throughout Europe so that organs are never wasted if they are physiologically and anatomically satisfactory.

After removal, organs such as kidneys, pancreas, liver and heart are cooled with special preservative solutions and transported to the recipient's hospital usually by simple surface cooling. It is now possible to transplant kidneys up to 24 hours after removal and there has been some success up to 48 hours. Other organs survive storage less well and are usually transplanted within 6 hours of removal.

On occasions it should be possible for a nurse looking after a hopeless head injury who is diagnosed brain dead to bring a chance of life to six other patients—a heart, a liver, a kidney and pancreas to a diabetic and a kidney—two more patients taking the vacated haemodialysis machines—a further two patients should regain sight by corneal grafting. This surely is a 'gift of life' in the true nursing tradition. What joy to the donor's relatives if success occurs with even some of these grafts to set against the bereavement.

Chapter 9
Intensive Care in a Children's Hospital

Nursing staff who deal with the care of sick children tend to become more emotionally involved with their patients than is the case in adult hospitals, and the need for an intensive care unit in a children's hospital may be questioned. However it is the author's belief that such a unit forms an essential part of a children's hospital, and it is reasonable to state the aims of an ICU. These may be defined as providing a facility whereby more space, staff and equipment for patient care is provided than is possible in the ordinary ward environment, and a service providing continuous observation of vital functions, and support of those functions more efficiently than is possible in the general ward.

Nursing staff who are properly trained and aware of their increased responsibilities are required to perform tasks which hitherto may have been considered the province of medical staff. They must be able to regulate the complex equipment to which the patient may be attached, and must also be able to interpret complex data with which they are furnished, and act in an intelligent and rapid way, based on logical reasoning, on data provided by the various monitoring devices.

'Monitoring' of a patient's vital functions requires some explanation. The nurse or junior doctor must not be 'mesmerized by machinery' so that monitoring (or measurement) becomes a recording of gradual deterioration of the patient's condition to a fatal termination. The reason for patient monitoring is to enable deviation from normal physiology, or more usually, deviations from the path of correction of abnormal physiology as it is being restored to normal, to be recognized early so that appropriate correction can be applied before serious life threatening complications have ensued.

A fundamental principle in intensive therapy is that all patients requiring the service should be grouped together, irrespective of

172

the nature of their disease, the only criterion for admission to an ICU being the severity of the disease process. Children, particularly young children and infants, who are ill are particularly prone to infection, while children with infections are susceptible to complications. The presence of infection must not be a bar to admission to the ICU and indeed may well be an indication for admission. Thus a child with a severe meningoencephalitis may well require support of his respiration, while an infant who has had major surgery may contract gastroenteritis. Provision for the nursing of such cases must be made by having cubicles within the unit and enforcing strict barrier nursing. A further important principle is that duplication of intensive care areas should be avoided, so that, for example, the hospital does not have a 'respiratory unit' and 'general ICU'. It is preferable that the ICU should be linked to some variety of medical or surgical practice, so that a reasonable work load can be ensured at all times and seasonal variation avoided (as occurs, for example, in a purely respiratory unit) which leads to periods of boredom and frustration in the nursing staff.

It is important to realize that infants and young children cannot be regarded as 'miniature adults', as they have important differences both in their normal physiology, and in the reaction of the body to disease. It is obviously impossible in this chapter to give more than a review of the problems encountered and further information should be obtained from books devoted to paediatric intensive care. It is difficult to provide statistical evidence that treatment of children in an intensive care ward saves lives, in view of the fact that any patient may pose problems which are not exactly similar to those of another patient with a similar clinical state. However, there is no doubt that such an environment does provide the most favourable conditions for survival in that continuous reassessment of the patient's condition, and correction of deviations from the normal course of recovery, are made with the minimum of delay.

The patients admitted to a paediatric ICU will vary in age from the newborn to the young teenager, and in general terms they may require special care because of:

1. The need to provide assistance to respiration, either because of respiratory disease, or because support is needed as a result of other conditions, such as cardiovascular operations, status epilepticus, poisoning, etc.

2. The need to maintain cardiovascular integrity.
3. The special care necessary in the patient who is unconscious, from a variety of causes.
4. The management of toxaemia.
5. The meticulous care necessary in treatment of acute renal failure.

The length of stay in the ICU will depend solely on the need for support of the patient's vital functions by mechanical or electronic means, or by virtue of detailed biochemical correction of disturbed physiology. The unit must *not* be used as a means of relieving a general ward of work because it may be relatively understaffed.

Certain features of paediatric care will now be discussed in more detail.

Fluid and electrolyte balance, and energy requirements

The major proportion of the body weight is due to water, but the distribution of body water in childhood presents important differences from that in the adult. Proportional to its size the infant has a greater total body water than the child and the child more so than the adult. The difference lies in the water contained between the cells of the body, that is, the interstitial fluid. At all ages water in the cells constitutes about 45% of body weight in kg, while plasma forms 5%, and whole blood 8%. The change with age occurs not in the vascular compartment but in the interstitial compartment; thus extracellular fluid up to the age of one month forms 30% of body weight, between one month and one year 25%, and from one year to twelve years 20%.

The balance of water and sodium in the body is closely related, and retention of one within the body usually implies retention of the other. Sodium is largely present outside the cells, whereas potassium is predominantly an intracellular ion, and is intimately linked with protein synthesis and breakdown, so that it is vitally important in the growing child. Normal water, sodium and potassium requirements vary with age. Thus the infant up to the age of one year (excluding the first week of life) requires water to the extent of 150 ml/kg of body weight, sodium and potassium each being 2.5 mmol/kg. It must be stressed that these are normal amounts, and may need to be increased or decreased according to deranged physiology; thus an infant in cardiac failure may require

some restriction of sodium and water intake, while in gastroenteritis there will be an increased requirement of water and electrolytes. Adrenocortical stimulation causes sodium (and therefore
water) retention and increased urinary excretion of potassium.
Drugs such as spironolactone block the effect of aldosterone on the
kidney and thus promote sodium (and therefore water) loss.

In the case of infants of low birth weight (less than 2.5 kg), who
may be either premature (judged by gestational date) or dysma-
ture (expected gestational date but 'small for dates'), water
requirement is significantly greater and should be estimated at
200 ml/kg body weight/24 hours.

As the child grows his maintenance needs of water and electrolytes decrease so that by the age of 7 years water is required in a
daily amount of 70 ml/kg of body weight, while sodium and potassium requirements are each 1.5 mmol/kg.

Water, sodium and potassium balance in the body depends on
intake and on losses. A pure water deficiency will result in dehydration, with a high serum sodium level—*hypernatraemia*—and a
child in this state will often appear deceptively well hydrated, as
the vascular compartment is not contracted. More usually both
water and sodium are depleted in dehydration, the serum sodium
being relatively normal (isotonic dehydration), and the clinical
appearance will vary according to the amount of water and sodium
deficit, from an irritable, slightly flushed child who is very thirsty
(mild dehydration, corresponding to a deficit of 15% of extracellular fluid), to an apathetic unresponsive child, with hypotonia,
staring sunken eyes and circulatory collapse (severe dehydration,
corresponding to a 30% deficit of extracellular fluid).

Hyponatraemia (a low serum sodium) may be found in true
sodium depletion where excessive losses of sodium have occurred;
in cardiac failure; in primary water overload; in inappropriate
secretion of the antidiuretic hormone by the pituitary, and in the
'sick cell' syndrome. The latter is of particular interest in ill children, and is due to failure of the 'sodium pump' mechanism of the
cell membrane so that sodium is lost from the extracellular fluid
into the cell and potassium leaks from the cell into the extracellular compartment. The mechanism is influenced by insulin secretion by the pancreas.

Potassium is mainly an intracellular ion, and is essential for
protein reconstruction and tissue synthesis. This is important in
considering breakdown of tissue due to trauma and disease, when

both potassium and nitrogen are lost from the body, the latter coming from the proteins. It has been estimated that a loss of 5 kg of muscle proteins requires 600 mmol of potassium together with the necessary protein nitrogen for its replacement.

Potassium depletion—*hypokalaemia*—tends to cause a metabolic alkalosis, and alkalosis predisposes to hypokalaemia. A potassium deficit causes impaired function of cardiac, skeletal and smooth muscle so that cardiac arrhythmias, muscular weakness and paralytic ileus may occur. *Hyperkalaemia*, in which the serum potassium is raised, may occur due to the sick cell syndrome, excessive intake (particularly if this is intravenous), and when potassium excretion is impaired (renal failure). The toxic effects are most severe in relation to cardiac action, and result eventually in complete heart block and ventricular fibrillation.

Disturbances of fluid and electrolyte balance can occur very quickly in small children, and require urgent correction before severe secondary effects have manifested themselves. Children must be reassessed at frequent intervals if they are receiving fluid and electrolyte solutions by intravenous infusion, and periodic serum electrolyte estimations must be done as frequently as deemed necessary, but certainly once every 24 hours. Serum sodium levels give a reasonably good reflection of total body sodium, but serum potassium levels (since potassium is mainly an intracellular ion) give only a very rough check. Daily weight recording is the best guide to fluctuations in the state of hydration, and it is also important from this point of view to measure urine output every twelve hours, recording each volume passed with a note of colour and specific gravity, together with biochemical assessment of the 24-hour excretion of electrolytes and urea.

Intravenous fluid and electrolyte therapy should be by per-cutaneous puncture rather than 'cut down' whenever possible, in order to spare veins, and scalp vein infusion sets are particularly useful in infants. Difficulties are experienced if conventional 'drip' sets are employed because of the small volumes of fluid to be infused in the smaller patients, and the tendency for the flow through fine canulae to cease when depending on a gravitational head of pressure. Some form of mechanical pressure infusor allowing accurate control of volumes is essential, such as the 'IMED' 922 Volumetric Infusor Pump.

In addition to fluid and electrolytes the sick child requires energy producing materials. Energy in the body is derived ultimately from the chemical energy of food (carbohydrates, fats and proteins), and the major output of energy by the body is in the form of heat. Chemical energy is required for the metabolic processes in the cells, electrical energy is produced by muscular contraction and neural activity, and mechanical energy is necessary for locomotion. As well as providing energy, proteins also furnish certain essential amino acids which are necessary for the construction of protein molecules, and are thus important in the context of repair of diseased or injured tissues. An adequate protein intake is also important for proper growth. Tissue protein undergoes a process of continual breakdown and re-synthesis, and this protein turnover means that nitrogen intake should balance nitrogen loss.

Relative to its size, the infant's energy requirement is much greater than the adult's. Thus the newborn needs 110 cals/kg/24 hours while by the age of 7 years the energy requirement has decreased to 70 cals/kg. In the case of infants of low birth weight the requirement is even greater, about 130 cals/kg. It is important to realise that in the hypercatabolic state resulting from disease or trauma the requirement will be considerably more than the 'normal' value during health.

Provided that the child has good renal function and is taking a balanced diet by mouth there is no problem in maintaining adequate nutrition in most patients. However, when disease or trauma cause interference with normal absorptive processes intravenous feeding is required. This presents serious difficulties in childhood and particularly in infancy. Prolonged intravenous infusions have a serious risk of bacterial or fungal infections. In addition to the fluid and electrolytes necessary, the intravenous infusion must provide calories in the form of carbohydrates (sugar solutions), fat emulsions and amino acids. The difficulty in the construction of an adequate intravenous régime lies in the fact that the total volume of fluid allowable is small, and that most of the amino acid solutions available contain fairly large amounts of sodium. Thus in order to give the correct amount of nitrogen as amino acid solution, one would usually have to give too much fluid and too much sodium. The excessive amount of sodium and water may be eliminated satisfactorily if renal function is good, but in most instances it is better to be guided by water and electrolyte requirements, and to be content with a less than optimum nitrogen intake. Fortunately, prolonged intravenous feeding is rarely necessary.

Respiratory problems in childhood

If the arterial PCO_2 is above normal, or the PO_2 is below normal, due to some condition affecting the lungs, then the patient is in respiratory failure. Conditions which may cause this in childhood include respiratory obstruction (upper or lower); depression of the respiratory centre (e.g. head injury, drug overdosage); limitation of movement of the thoracic cage (e.g. diaphragm splinted by gross abdominal distension); compression of the lung (e.g. pleural effusion); and pulmonary disease resulting in decrease of functioning lung tissue (e.g fibrocystic disease) or decreased compliance (pulmonary vascular congestion secondary to congenital heart disease).

Blood gas determinations are essential in the diagnosis of respiratory failure and in checking the effects of treatment. Arterial blood is preferable, but there is a limit to the number of arterial punctures that should be performed on small vessels with the risk of complications such as infection and thrombosis, so that capillary blood may be used, providing it is taken from a warm vasodilated heel or finger. Gas measurements on blood taken after great pressure from a vasoconstricted area, when peripheral circulatory failure is present, are useless and misleading.

In every case of respiratory failure in childhood obvious causes (such as a foreign body or the compression of the lung by a diaphragmatic hernia) should be sought and treated. Infections, if sensitive to antibiotics, should be treated with the appropriate one, but, in infancy particularly, severe respiratory distress may be due to viral infections for which antibiotics are of little value except in an attempt to reduce or prevent secondary bacterial invasion.

In general terms the treatment of respiratory failure in childhood should follow certain fundamental principles. A close watch must be kept on pulse and respiratory rate, the general appearance (presence of intercostal recession, use of accessory muscles of respiration, colour, presence of sweating, etc.) and the temperature, in addition to the repeated blood gas estimations. Intercostal recession is the indrawing of the spaces between the ribs during inspiration. Sometimes the whole of the lower rib cage and upper abdomen is sucked inwards as well.

A child who is fretful and restless is usually so because of hypoxia and his restlessness causes a worsening of the situation because of greater oxygen consumption; cautious sedation is necessary, but continuing restlessness is *not* an indication for further sedation but may well mean that support to respiration must be given.

The air passages of children are small, and infants are particularly at risk because the airway is critically situated between adequate and obstructed. Since the resistance to flow through the airway varies as the fourth power of the radius, the presence of only a thin layer of sticky exudate can severely distress an infant. Adequate humidification of inspired gas is thus mandatory, and may be by aerosol nebulization of water into an incubator or plastic tent, or by use of an ultrasonic nebulizer. The latter must be used with caution particularly in infants because of the danger of water overload. It is important to keep the patient well hydrated to prevent thickening of tracheobronchial secretions. Dehydration is soon followed by crusting of secretions in the air passages.

Respiratory stimulants such as nikethamide should *never* be used. They are non-specific cerebral stimulants, they increase oxygen need, and their effect lasts for a much shorter time than the disease process. They may cause convulsions especially in the hypoxic patient.

Oxygen should be given if necessary, but only enough to improve arterial oxygen saturation. A high intake damages the lungs, and in the newborn can produce retrolental fibroplasia, leading to blindness.

If the above measures fail to produce improvement, intubation of the trachea is necessary, preferably under general anaesthesia to avoid trauma. In an emergency an oral endotracheal tube is used, but for long-term use an oral tube tends to be unstable and may be bitten by the patient, so either a Jackson Rees nasotracheal tube (see Fig. 39) is employed or a tracheostomy is done. Nasotracheal intubation can be used for about five days in the child, or ten days in the infant, and if the artificial airway is necessary for longer than this a tracheostomy should be done. While the Björk type of 'tracheal flap' tracheostomy is satisfactory in older children, as tube changing is easy and incorrect positioning of the tube is unlikely to occur, its use in infants and small children may be followed by forward angulation of the trachea kinking it and making eventual decannulation difficult or impossible. In such infants a 'slit' tracheostomy is preferable, but aftercare must be meticulous until a good track has formed since accidental displacement of the tube may result in severe respiratory obstruction.

Plastic disposable tracheostomy tubes are preferable, as they cause minimal irritation of the respiratory tract epithelium. For infants the Great Ormond Street pattern tube (see Fig. 39) is particularly useful as it has a wide lumen at the flange, so allowing easy use of endotracheal connectors for hand inflation and connection to a ventilator. Whatever means of bypassing the nose and pharynx are employed, the natural humidification mechanism is lost, so that humidification of the inspired gas by artificial means becomes even more important.

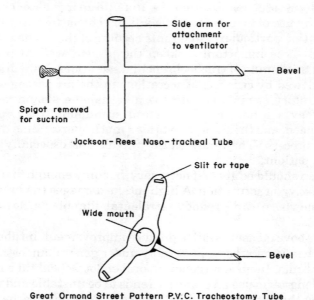

Fig. 39. Tubes to connect infants to ventilators.

Bronchial lavage may be necessary to loosen tracheobronchial secretions, small amounts of sterile normal saline being employed. After lavage and suction the lungs should be hand inflated through a rebreathing bag and endotracheal connector attached to an oxygen line. Failure to do this will result in multiple small areas of collapse throughout the lungs, with the production of a right-to-left shunt and further arterial oxygen desaturation.

If respiratory failure persists artificial ventilation of the lungs will be necessary. This has its own complications and must not lightly be undertaken in childhood. Several types of intermittent positive pressure machines are available and the machine and circuit appropriate for the patient's condition and size must be carefully selected. Children being assisted with a ventilator require adequate sedation, and probably diazepam is the most useful tranquillizing agent. If there is a strong respiratory drive causing tachypnoea, a respiratory depressant such as phenoperidine, or a muscle-relaxant like alcuronium will be necessary.

A few of the conditions which may require artificial ventilation in childhood will now be outlined.

1. Respiratory distress syndrome of the newborn. This is associated with prematurity and possible lack of surfactant. Progressive respiratory difficulty occurs between soon after birth and the third day of life, with rib recession, cyanosis and expiratory grunting. The earlier the onset the less likely is there to be a successful outcome.

2. Respiratory inadequacy in infants of very low birth weight (less than 1.5 kg) may range from periods of hypoventilation with episodes of apnoea, to the Wilson-Mikity syndrome of respiratory insufficiency, with a lacy reticulation of the lungs on radiography between the second and third week, which may improve or progress to emphysema, cyst formation or fibrosis.

3. Virus bronchiolitis. This usually begins as a cold, which is followed by increasing dyspnoea and rib recession, with the production of overdistended lungs due to bronchospasm.

4. Acid aspiration syndrome (Mendelson). This is due to the inhalation of acid gastric contents causing severe oedema and spasm of the bronchioles. If untreated, or if there is no response to treatment, death may occur due to pulmonary oedema and bronchopneumonia.

5. Pulmonary vascular congestion. This may be due to congenital heart disease with left-to-right shunt, and the increased pulmonary blood flow causes decreased compliance with 'stiff' lungs. Artificial ventilation may be necessary prior to and also subsequent to operative treatment for the underlying condition.

The use of continuous positive airways pressure, in which the pressure in the bronchial tree is always maintained above atmospheric pressure, has many advantages. The lungs are not inflated mechanically, but the endotracheal tube is connected by a 'T' piece to an oxygen/air supply and to a tube which is placed so that its end is 5 to 10 cm below the surface of aqueous hibitane in a bottle. An antifoam agent is added (see Fig. 40). In order to bubble out of the end of this tube, gas pressures in the system must exceed 5–10 cmH$_2$O. The gentle inflation of the lungs so obtained is a useful intermediate stage in weaning the child from mechanical ventilation; it is of benefit in the respiratory distress syndrome, pulmonary oedema and when air passages have lost their rigidity and tend to collapse on inspiration.

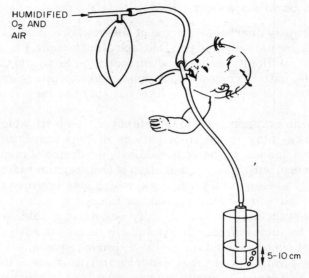

HUMIDIFIED
O$_2$ AND
AIR

5–10 cm

Fig. 40. Apparatus for continuous positive airways pressure.

Some infants do not necessarily require endotracheal intubation to raise the airway pressure as a sufficient assistance to ventilation can be achieved by using the same system attached to an indwelling short nasopharyngeal tube. This is also useful as a means of weaning from endotracheal intubation with continuous positive pressure.

Cardiovascular problems

Broadly speaking, children suffering from congenital heart defects have abnormalities in the circulation because of simple obstructions to the flow of blood, communications between the systemic and pulmonary circulation, valvular insufficiencies, and combinations of the above.

From the point of view of ICU management, the effects of the deranged anatomy will be shown as an abnormal work load on one or other ventricle or both, or the production of chronic hypoxia and its complications, or to increased difficulty in breathing due to decreased pulmonary compliance. Treatment of congenital heart disease is essentially a simple concept, the ideal being the restoration of normal physiology by the correction of the anatomical defects. Some operations are done using conventional techniques, others require the use of cardiopulmonary bypass.

The necessity for post-operative care in an ICU depends on the pre-operative state of the patient; on the complexity of the operation and on the likelihood of serious post-operative difficulties. Thus the routine interruption of a persistent ductus arteriosus is not likely to necessitate an ICU stay, whereas the same operation, done as a semi-emergency procedure for an infant in heart failure, is likely to be followed by a post-operative period of some anxiety, and indeed mechanical assistance to ventilation may be necessary.

After a complex heart operation the nurse must be able to record data, while a constant watch must be kept on the electrocardiogram monitored on an oscilloscope. In addition to recordings of temperature, pulse and respiration and sphygmomanometer cuff measurement of systolic arterial pressure, indwelling cannulae are inserted at operation for measurement of:

1. Central venous or right atrial pressure
2. Systemic arterial pressure
3. Usually, left atrial pressure

The reason for recording arterial pressure both directly and by sphygmomanometer lies in the fact that these two readings do not coincide. The direct intra-arterial pressure is the 'correct' one, but it is useful to have a 'cuff' pressure as well to provide a base line for the time when the arterial line is withdrawn. The arterial cannula is also of use in providing samples of blood for acid-base studies, blood-gas determinations, electrolyte and other biochemical determinations.

In view of the small calibre of the recording cannulae patency of these must be ensured by periodic flushing with a little heparinized saline.

Where chronic hypoxia has been present before operation the response of the body is to increase red cell and haemoglobin production so that the patient becomes polycythaemic. This has the advantage to the patient that the oxygen carrying capacity of the blood is increased, but a serious disadvantage is that the blood viscosity is also increased (with consequent increased cardiac work) and the patient is at risk from spontaneous intravascular thrombosis especially if the cardiac output falls or if he becomes dehydrated. It is thus imperative in the post-operative patient to maintain a good cardiac output with good peripheral perfusion, and to ensure that adequate hydration is present without however giving an excessive fluid load with the risk of producing cardiac failure. Haematocrit determination and central venous pressure recordings are extremely useful in assessing both the state of hydration and the ability of the right ventricle to cope with the infused fluid.

When there has been obstruction of either ventricle operative relief of the obstruction may be followed by some degree of ventricular failure. On the right side this will be manifested by a rise of central venous pressure, enlargement of the liver, and systemic venous oedema, and supportive treatment will include measures to improve cardiac function and to eliminate excess water and sodium. Failure of the left ventricle, shown by a rise of left atrial pressure, results in pulmonary oedema which again requires measures to improve the working of the left ventricle and eliminate salt and water, but in this instance the accumulation of fluid between and in the alveoli leads to a progressive decrease in pulmonary compliance, for which mechanical ventilation of the lungs may be essential; positive pressure ventilation of the lungs is employed, some mechanism being used to give an end expiratory pressure of between 5 and 10 cmH$_2$O.

Left to right shunts which have been satisfactorily treated surgically may produce difficulties after operation for two reasons. Firstly, if a high pulmonary blood flow has been present pre-operatively the presence of 'stiff' lungs post-operatively, together with restriction of breathing due to pain, will produce some degree of respiratory failure (rise in arterial PCO$_2$, fall in PO$_2$) sufficient to require mechanical ventilation. Secondly, if the left-to-right shunt has resulted in severe changes in the pulmonary vascular bed, so that resistance to flow of blood is greatly increased, after the shunt has been obliterated at operation the unsupported right ventricle may fail causing severe congestive failure needing energetic medical treatment.

After any cardiac operation attention must be directed to assessing cardiac output and to maintaining this if the pump begins to fail. Pump failure, resulting in impaired tissue perfusion, will cause a metabolic acidosis with a lowering of pH and a lowering of the standard bicarbonate. Although it is easy, and indeed necessary, to restore the pH to near normal by giving sodium bicarbonate intravenously, this does not cure the cause of the acidosis, and measures must be adopted to improve cardiac function and tissue perfusion.

Cardiac output may be impaired because of insufficient blood transfusion, compression of the heart by inadequate pericardial drainage, hypoxia and acidosis, electrolyte disturbances, and disturbance of cardiac rhythm or rate. If the above have been eliminated as a cause of low output this may be due to 'pump failure' and supportive therapy involves the use of drugs to improve cardiac action. Noradrenaline, which increases blood pressure by constricting peripheral vessels, should not be used as it *increases* the work to be done by a failing pump. Adrenaline increases stroke output and heart rate, but has the disadvantage of constricting skin vessels and the renal vascular bed. Isoprenaline primarily acts by increasing cardiac rate, and also has a peripheral vasodilating action. In therapeutic doses dopamine increases stroke output without too much increase in rate and vasoconstriction. In practice combinations of these 'catecholamine' type drugs may be used, and frequently thymoxamine is added to the drug or drugs given in order to promote peripheral and renal vasodilation. Such drugs *must* be given in carefully controlled doses with minimum fluid through a central venous cannula, and an infusor pump such as the Vickers Medical 'TREONIC IP3' Digital Syringe Pump is essential.

Heart block may have arisen as a result of trauma to the conducting tissue of the heart, and may be managed by direct pacing via leads inserted into the myocardium at operation.

In very major cardiac reconstructive operations with low cardiac output it may be necessary to give a high venous plasma load in order to achieve satisfactory whole body perfusion. Unfortunately, the kidneys do not always cope with this and an outpouring of fluid into the peritoneal cavity (ascites) may necessitate peritoneal drainage, as the increased intraperitoneal pressure interferes with pulmonary ventilation and venous returns to the heart (so lowering cardiac output).

If low cardiac output is associated with oliguria or anuria with no response to diuretic therapy within the first 12 hours after operation, peritoneal dialysis should be instituted *even if there is no great electrolyte (mainly potassium) disturbance*, because the main problem is retention of water which will affect gas exchange in the lungs, leading to acidosis, and this will decrease cardiac output.

The neonate in the ICU

The neonate is particularly at risk for several reasons:

1. The temperature regulating mechanism is unstable so that he is very dependent on the temperature of his environment; thus he can easily either overheat or become hypothermic.
2. The airway is critically small so that airway obstruction is readily provoked by drying of bronchial secretions.
3. Defence mechanisms to microbial invasion are not yet efficient, so that a severe infection is liable to be followed by septicaemia. Moreover, broad spectrum antibiotic therapy may leave the path open to systemic invasion by monilia.
4. While the infant's kidney can handle water satisfactorily, there is evidence that sodium excretion continues despite body sodium depletion.
5. The central nervous system is unstable, and insults to it (e.g. hyperpyrexia, water intoxication, hypoxia) are not infrequently accompanied by convulsions.

Since loss of body heat occurs so readily many sick infants are nursed in incubators, this having the advantage that warmth, humidity and an oxygen enriched atmosphere can all be provided. Generalized humidity has some disadvantage in that an environment is provided which is favourable to the growth of *Ps. pyocyanea*. Contamination of the incubator by the infant's excreta is another factor to be considered in relation to infection so that frequent changes of incubator are necessary to allow of effective sterilization (e.g. every 48 hours). While added oxygen may be necessary in the treatment of hypoxia, care must be taken not to exceed optimum concentrations because of the danger of producing retrolental fibroplasia, and perhaps oxygen damage to the lungs although this uncommon complication is more usually seen if artificial ventilation of the lungs is being employed.

Since thickening of bronchial secretions must be prevented it is often useful to employ humidified inspired gas led into a miniature plastic tent around the baby's head. Great care must be taken if an ultrasonic nebulizer is used because of the danger of water overload.

All technical manipulations (airway suction, setting up an intravenous infusion etc.) should be done as aseptically as possible because of the risk of infection. This often means the use of two nurses to treat one baby. Regular bacteriological investigation is necessary in management (e.g. tracheal suction catheters after aspirating the airway, pharyngeal or umbilical bacteriological swabs etc.) but only if an organism is producing ill-health should it be treated with antibiotics, otherwise the path may be opened to invasion by antibiotic resistant bacteria or fungi.

Undue handling of an infant is to be avoided so that he is allowed adequate rest, but rest should not mean dimming of lights so that adequate observation is not possible. The infant can sleep quite satisfactorily with full illumination. If oral feeding is not possible, or is obviously tiring the infant, he should be tube fed. The only certain indication that a feeding tube is in the stomach is by radiological proof, so that feeding tubes should have a radio-opaque strip marker along their length.

Some problems which may be met include:

1. Oesophageal atresia. In this condition the infant cannot swallow his saliva and is thus at risk from inhalation pneumonia. Treatment is therefore essentially directed to relieving the oesophageal obstruction, either by doing an oesophageal anastomosis, in which case feeding can soon take place via an indwelling nasogastric tube, or by draining the upper oesophagus on to the surface of the neck and feeding the child via a gastrostomy. Most of these infants also have a communication between the lower oesophagus and the trachea (tracheo-oesophageal fistula) which must be obliterated in order to avoid the risk of gastro-tracheal regurgitation with inhalation of acid gastric juice. Many of the infants have respiratory complications (lobar collapse, rib recession, etc.) at the time of admission, and post-operative management is largely directed to the maintenance of good lung function.

2. Jaundice. Some degree of jaundice occurs in all newborn infants and does not necessarily indicate rhesus or ABO incompatability between the baby and his mother, but reflects the fact that the liver is not yet able to cope adequately with the bile pigment resulting from the normal destruction of red cells. However, jaundice should be carefully watched with daily estimations of serum bilirubin, as levels exceeding 20 mg may cause brain damage (kernicterus) and may be an indication for exchange transfusion whatever the cause of the jaundice. Other causes of jaundice are prematurity, bacterial infection, hypothyroidism, galactosaemia, hepatitis and atresia of the bile ducts. It must be remembered that any of these may complicate the condition for which the infant was admitted to the ICU.

3. Diaphragmatic hernia. The infant who is admitted with this condition is in severe respiratory distress due to a mass of intestines filling one pleural cavity, compressing the lung, and pushing the heart and mediastinum to the opposite side so interfering with function of the other lung. The pressure of the intestines in the chest before birth causes interference with growth of the lung. After operation such infants may continue to have respiratory difficulties because the lung (sometimes both lungs) is small and underdeveloped, and also because the diaphragm may be splinted with a mass of intestines crammed into an abdominal cavity which is really not large enough to accommodate them. In these circumstances oral or tube feeding is contra-indicated until good bowel function is established, and assisted ventilation may be necessary.

4. Cardiac problems. Most infants who are admitted to an ICU with heart disease will have been operated on in an attempt to help cardiac failure by improving oxygenation, or decreasing a left-to-right shunt, or by decreasing excessive left ventricular work due to coarctation of the aorta. In the first week or so of life hypoxia due to heart disease is likely to be due to the Fallot variety of defect, or to transposition of the great arteries. Where pulmonary blood flow is reduced, as in the baby with tetralogy of Fallot, an aorta-pulmonary shunt gives the best chance of survival. The palliation of transposition of the great arteries depends on getting adequate mixing of right and left atrial blood by the creation of an atrial septal defect either in the catheterization laboratory (balloon septostomy) or in the operating theatre (Blalock-Hanlon operation). In both of these cyanotic conditions there is usually a severe metabolic acidosis requiring correction, while care must be taken to watch kidney function and also to prevent dehydration.

Left-to-right shunts are treated where possible by curative procedures (e.g. ligation of a persistent ductus arteriosus) but if these are not possible pulmonary blood flow is reduced to manageable proportions by pulmonary artery banding. Following banding the pulmonary compliance may improve fairly rapidly, but if ventilatory difficulties persist a period of artificial ventilation of the lungs may be necessary.

Coarction of the aorta requiring treatment in infancy is always accompanied by some other cardiac defect (e.g. ventricular septal defect), and the indication for surgical treatment is cardiac failure which does not rapidly respond to medical management. The pulmonary compliance is always reduced and post-operative ventilation of the lungs by machine is frequently necessary.

Chapter 10
'The Patient is a Person'

It would not be surprising if the reader had by now gained the impression that intensive care nursing is a coldly scientific calling. It may well seem that the rather complex technical skills demanded could only be carried out by an impersonal technician. It may seem to be a far cry from the ideals which attracted you to nursing in the first place. Most of us do not mind working ourselves into the ground if our efforts are appreciated. Nurses like doctors, find the relationship with their patients to be one of the most rewarding aspects of their work. Unfortunately, many of the patients nursed in an intensive care unit are so sick that they may be incapable of appreciating all that is being done for them and indeed many will tell you when they are well again that they have no recollection of having been in the intensive care unit at all. The ICU nurse may feel that, although it is her work which has put the patient on the road to recovery, it is the ward nurse who gets the boxes of chocolates.

It is all too easy to come to regard your unresponsive patient as a bundle of physiological systems which have to be measured, charted and forced to conform to the state which we have come to regard as normal. Where there is no apparent need for a bedside manner the bed can very easily become a laboratory bench. In fact nothing could be further from the truth than the concept that the patient is too sick to require the encouragement, kindness and consolation which only a nurse can give, but it can sometimes be difficult to maintain this human approach. A kind of compassion is demanded of the type which is all too familiar to those who have to nurse the mentally handicapped.

Just consider for a moment the stresses which a patient in an intensive care unit may have to undergo. He is in unfamiliar surroundings, and probably does not know the nurses about him. He may be in pain and will almost certainly be very frightened. It

190

will be difficult to sleep because the lights are always on and even if he is not being roused to have his blood pressure taken or be given an injection, the constant activity in other parts of the unit will be a continuous disturbance. He is surrounded by blinking lights, oscilloscope screens and squeaking cardiac monitors. The monotonous chug of the ventilator becomes an additional torment. To crown all this he may be unable to communicate and share his fears because he has an endotracheal tube in his throat. The constant illumination blends day into night and the absence of such familiar landmarks as breakfast, lunch and tea destroys all sense of time. This is a disturbing catalogue which may have a familiar ring about it, for the circumstances are almost exactly those used in brainwashing and the more sophisticated forms of torture. It is small wonder that mental disturbance and hallucinations are common. Some doctors who care very deeply about their patients have said that the terrors of intensive care should not be inflicted on anyone and there is much to sympathize with in this point of view. However, there is no dispute that intensive care can be life-saving. Many patients are now alive who would otherwise certainly have died without the benefits of intensive care and without it many of the new and valuable techniques in medicine and surgery would be impossible. Intensive care can be made tolerable for the patient if doctors and nurses will put themselves into the patient's position and exercise a little thoughtfulness.

Let us consider each of the unpleasant aspects of intensive care in turn and see what can be done to make them tolerable. Pain can be treated with any one of the wide range of drugs available. The best way of administering the more potent drugs such as morphia or omnopon has been suggested in Chapter 4 but quite often less powerful preparations will be adequate. Although the responsibility for prescribing analgesics rests with the doctor, the nurse has a duty to decide when they need to be administered and the patient may not be able to tell her that he is in pain. You will have to make a point of asking the patient directly at fairly frequent intervals and exercise a certain amount of common sense for the patient who is paralysed and on a ventilator.

Sleeplessness presents a rather more difficult problem. The unit should be designed so that the strong lights are not directly over the patient's head as he lies on his back. A compromise must be reached between the patient's comfort and the need for continuous observation. Lights have been designed which are capable of being

dimmed or tilted so that they shine away from the head of the bed.
A simple eye-shade can be very effective. It is to be hoped that the
use of devices which record the blood pressure continuously will
eventually replace the sphygmomanometer cuff. The many sedative drugs available can be remarkably effective and allow the
patient to have an adequate amount of sleep. Make sure that these
are prescribed for your patient. Oddly enough, many patients who
have been managed on a ventilator have no recollection of having
been in the unit at all. This is because the PCO_2 in a ventilated
patient is often lower than normal and produces a rather hazy,
dreamy state.

It is the management of fear that calls for the deepest patience
and understanding. It is helpful, although not always possible in
the busy and understaffed unit, for some member of the staff to
visit the patient before his operation and explain something of
what he is to expect. It will also serve to enable the nurse to get
some idea of the patient's character. Beware of the patient who is
overcheerful or who protests that he is not frightened of anything.
Some fear is only natural. We have found from a study of patients
undergoing open heart surgery that it is just those patients who
seem to be unnaturally brave or lighthearted who are most likely
to develop psychological disorders in the unit. It goes without
saying that the patient should as far as possible be told what is
going on. Ignorance is a very large part of fear. It is equally
important never to let the patient overhear any gloomy prophesy
about his future and above all not to discuss his progress across the
bed as if he were not there. Even though the patient may appear to
be unconscious his auditory nerves may be functioning as any
anaesthetist will tell you. There have been instances when a
patient has been able to repeat a conversation between the
surgeons in the operating theatre although he was apparently
asleep at the time. Strangely, despite being able to hear quite well
he will not have been aware of any pain.

It is important to avoid anxiety in the coronary care unit. If
possible patients should be isolated from each other by screens or
partitions. The same holds true for any intensive care unit.
Nothing could be more disturbing than to be the witness of cardiac
massage being performed on the patient in the next bed—but such
things do happen. Modern tranquillizer drugs can do much to allay
a patient's anxieties and we have found diazepam (Valium) and
chlordiazepoxide (Librium) to be very effective.

The practice of nursing men and women together is prevalent and usually patients are too ill to be disturbed by this, but as they recover it would not be unreasonable to make a few concessions to modesty. One's dignity is very precious. Once again, put yourself in the patient's position.

We have already discussed the need for providing some means of communication for patients with an indwelling endotracheal tube or a tracheostomy. A note pad, a pencil and a handbell are usually sufficient. Quite remarkable achievements are possible with the aid of modern technology. We have cared for a young woman paralysed by myaesthenia gravis who was unable to move any part of her body save the big toe on one foot. With this she was able to operate a machine which changed the station on her radio and operated a typewriter. Lastly, do not forget if you are nursing children, how reassuring a familiar object such as a doll or a teddy bear can be.

Almost as important as the nurse's relationship with the patient, are her dealings with the patient's relatives. Not unnaturally they will be extremely anxious. Restricted visiting once a day and the occasional comment over the telephone that the patient is 'as well as can be expected' are scarcely reassuring. We allow unrestricted visiting and have set aside a room close to the unit which is equipped with a divan bed, chairs, magazines and the means for making tea. If you have been a patient yourself, you will know that prolonged visiting is a strain both on the patient and the visitor. Conversation soon dries up, as the patient's only concern is with the little world about him and all too often the visit lapses into an awkward silence with frequent glances at the clock. Try and let the relatives visit for a few minutes at fairly frequent intervals whenever there is a slack period in your nursing activities and do try to warn them of what they may see. It can be a great shock to see one's loved ones festooned with tubes and connected to a mass of impressive electrical equipment. Try to explain simply what is being done and emphasize that it is only for a short time. It is important that the relatives should be lead to understand that, although they are welcome in the unit and that every effort will be made to accommodate them, they are not under an obligation to remain within call day and night. Many have commitments to children or other dependants at home and it is a little unfair to add a feeling of guilt because they are not constantly at the bedside to their natural anxiety about the patient. There are times when you can say: 'Why not go home for a few hours' sleep, we will let you know if there is any change.'

This book cannot be regarded as a complete text of intensive care. It is a growing specialty, constantly incorporating new knowledge and entering new fields. The authors hope that these few chapters will be of some help to the nurse entering upon this most demanding and at the same time most rewarding branch of nursing.

Index